GO-Diet
The Goldberg-O'Mara Diet Plan

D0875145

GO-Diet

The Goldberg-O'Mara Diet Plan
The Key to Weight Loss and Healthy Eating

Jack Goldberg, Ph.D. and Karen O'Mara, D.O.

GO Corp

GO-Diet
The Goldberg-O'Mara Diet Plan
The Key to Weight Loss and Healthy Eating

Jack Goldberg, Ph.D. and Karen O'Mara, D.O.

GO-Diet, The Goldberg-O'Mara Diet Plan.
Copyright © 1999 Jack M. Goldberg and Karen O'Mara.
Printed and bound in the United States of America.
All rights reserved
Published by
GO Corp
P.O. Box 48026
Niles, IL 60714   90

E-Mail go_diet@hotmail.com
Web Page http://www.go-diet.com

ISBN # 0-9670846-0-1
Library of Congress Catalog Number: 99-94264

Dedication

This book is dedicated to over 50% of the US adult population who are struggling with their weight and the medical complications resulting from it. Hopefully, this will offer a first step.

Here is what people have written about the GO-Diet.

"I highly recommend this diet, and I believe on this diet I will finally make my goals. I have tried so many diets that I have lost track of the numbers. Again, thanks for making this diet available." J.S.

"Before going on the diet, I was forever gulping Maalox, tagamet, Zantac, etc. Acid reflux was a daily event, sometimes choking me in the middle of the night. I was constantly burping and otherwise. I had to avoid cucumbers, onions, hot spices, and sauerkraut lest I go into major gastrointestinal distress. I was treated with prescription tagamet earlier this year. I had to be very very careful of what I ate. Amazingly, since I've been on the GO-diet, I have been able to eat anything I want, whenever I want it. I have the constitution I had when I was 17 years old." C.K.

"Dear Drs. Goldberg and O'Mara,
I don't know if the words "Thank You" adequately express the gratitude I feel. I hope you realize the magnitude of your outstanding work."
    "The diet is so easy and takes care of most of your cravings. So far we are very happy on it and hope to make it a lifestyle change instead of a diet." J.S.

"Again thanks for opening my eyes to a different way to eat. I have seen significant health benefits, and have passed a copy of the GO Diet to at least 10 people." T.S.

"I want to thank you for your diet. I have lost 17 pounds in 3 months. That is about all I need to lose. I am 70 years old and plan to continue the program." M.H.

"Let me say I love your diet. I was never overweight, but I have lost 12 pounds and got down to 13% body fat. My LDL cholesterol has gone down and my HDL has gone up on this diet." D.D.

"I not only have lost weight, but I like myself again when I look in the mirror. I feel younger, more energetic and if I dare say sexier!!" D.G.

"Your diet is effortless and it really works! I just turned 50 and cannot go through the rest of my life heavy. I am motivated, encouraged and losing weight." L.S.

"After years of trying low-fat diets, eating and feeling unsatisfied, going off diets and regaining more weight, we feel this diet is very livable." M.U.

Foreword

by Berry Lewis, MD

When Dr. O'Mara asked if I would share my experiences with the **Goldberg-O'Mara Diet**, I agreed although it was not without some reservations. I've always been a "big guy" having played high school and college football, and like most ex-athletes, I remained active by playing basketball. However, like most, I was still under the misconception that I could eat as if I was years younger. Then two years ago, after a major knee injury resulting in a four hour operation and six weeks in a long leg cast, my weight ballooned to three hundred and twenty-five pounds. It was also during this time that I decided to quit smoking.

After spending the last year agonizing over how to control my weight, I decided to try their new diet. I had experimented with a few diets in the past although I am by no means a "diet fanatic" and was unsuccessful. Yet, none of the other diets that I had attempted changed my life like this one did. As the transition period quickly passed, I soon learned to count carbohydrates instead of calories and I learned to cook a variety of low carbohydrate dishes that my entire family could enjoy. By avoiding rice, pasta, and bread, I found myself eating all of the foods that I desired and was surprised to discover that the pounds began to come off and stay off.

One amazing discovery while I was in the early phases of this diet was that I was never hungry. Because, though restricting my carbohydrate intake, I was still able to eat enough food to be full and satisfied. One of the benefits of lowering one's insulin level is that you find that you don't have the fluctuations in your appetite or cravings. And subsequently, I now eat even smaller portions that before. It helps that I like fish and chicken, grilled meats and an occasional lean steak as well as the daily nuts and yogurt. And my cholesterol level remains virtually unchanged (it was 168 when I started this diet and is still 167 now).

This year I lost more than 75 pounds and 12 inches off my waist. But more important to me is the change in my self image, my self esteem, and my overall physical health. As a result, I have changed my target weight twice and now have a new target weight. This diet has proven to me that I can achieve whatever weight I choose in a reasonable time frame without suffering. My hope is that you too will be able to enjoy this diet, without reservations regarding counting calories or feeling hungry. Don't be afraid to experiment with new recipes and making your own foods (in the low carbohydrate way, of course!). And, begin to enjoy helping yourself and your family to appreciate a healthier, lower carbohydrate lifestyle.

Contents

Introduction

"You're fat because you eat too much and you don't exercise enough. Why don't you control yourself? Don't you have any self respect?" How often have you heard those words? Unfortunately for too many people, those questions are all too familiar.

Could this be you?

"I was downright skinny as a child, normal or chubby as an adolescent and trim as a young adult. But I have a family history of obesity. They weren't always fat. It seemed that about age 40 the weight started to appear and by their mid-to-late fifties, most of the people on my mother's side had developed Type 2 diabetes or heart trouble and all the medical problems that follow such as kidney disease and eyesight problems. Generally their last few years of life were no bed of roses.

"At age forty, I was 8 pounds heavier than I was at age twenty. I was also a smoker. At age forty-two I weighed one hundred and seventy two pounds and I gave up smoking cold turkey. That was December 2, 1986. By the following Christmas I weighed one hundred and ninety two pounds. My cholesterol was 240 mg/dL and my HDL cholesterol was a miserable 29 mg/dL."

That is the biographical information on one of the authors of this book. For the other, it was a history of weight gain after age 40, despite adherence to the Food Pyramid and low fat foods. Yet if we were doing the right things, why were we gaining weight and ending up with abnormal lab studies? Certainly we knew better, didn't we?

Not only had we failed ourselves, but as clinicians, we offered little of value to patients who turned to us for medical guidance with their diseases. In fact, we tended to fall into the same stereotyping of overweight people as the general public. They were fat because they were noncompliant with the diets we had given them. Of course, anyone reading this book knows what they were offered to lose weight: low fat, calorie-restricted diets. The same type of diet we ourselves were struggling with and gaining weight on.

Some may have resorted to prescription or over-the-counter diet pills, others to endless miles on treadmills, still others to bizarre diets that bore no relationship to normal foods. The results were the same regardless of the method. In the majority of cases, one saw some initial weight loss but usually of inconsequential amounts, and loss that was not sustained. Yet, also as clinicians, we knew we had a responsibility to look inward. If our prescriptions were so good, then why had there been a 30% increase in obesity in the United States in just the last 10 years? Was it right to keep blaming the victim or did we have a responsibility to improve our treatments, to directly face the presumptions we in medicine had about weight gain? When diets failed in the 45 year old woman, was it right to keep telling her that it was related to her hormones or that her metabolism was just slowing down? When ex-smokers turned to us in frustration because of weight gain, was it right to tell them just to eat less?

In 1996, with personal and professional frustrations high, we collaborated in an in-depth review of the scientific literature concerning weight loss and improvement in serum lipids through diet. We also looked at all of the popular diets being touted at the time. Although no one was ideal, we found there were often some selected aspects of each diet that were noteworthy. Indeed, any diet at the beginning may cause a little bit of weight loss. After all, you want to make it work, so maybe regardless of what it is you're advised to eat, you try to restrict the amount even further to get some weight loss. But what we were looking for was something that would result in consistent weight loss without deleterious effects on the rest of the metabolism and physiology of the body.

Looking at the subspecialty literature allowed us to find clinical trials that tested single dietary components in patients who already had diseases that were made worse by obesity. Slowly we extracted enough information to conclude that low carbohydrates in the diet could result in weight loss. But that was not enough to build a diet upon. What about the rest of the dietary components, fats and proteins, and macro-and micro-nutrients? The diabetes literature showed us that the use of high monounsaturated fats in the diet was associated with improved glucose control, especially in obese subjects. The preventative medicine literature discussed the importance of natural sources of vitamins, phytochemicals, and fiber. Things were coming together. We took elements of the best we had learned from the literature, the most rational data, and created **The Goldberg-O'Mara Diet for Weight Loss and Healthy Eating**. What we created was a diet that emphasizes very low carbohydrates with normal protein amounts, using high monounsaturated fats and reducing saturated fats, encouraging fiber, natural sources of vitamins and nutrients from a variety of vegetables and fermented milk products.

As conscientious scientists, we first used ourselves as subjects. Dr. Goldberg initiated the diet and lost 12 pounds in the first month. Dr. O'Mara started just before Halloween in 1996 and was 25 pounds lighter by Christmas. Our own laboratory studies confirmed its safety in the two of us. We were badgered for the diet and started our formal clinical studies in moderate-to-severely obese adult subjects in May, 1997. We and others have now used this diet more informally in hundreds of people of varying weights and ages.

The Goldberg-O'Mara Diet, and the data supporting its use, are now available for you. It's easy to follow and will become a way of life Try it for three months. It's just three months of a lifetime but it could change your life forever. If you respond to the diet like the average moderate-to-severely obese subject in our study, you may see the average weight loss of 20 pounds, a drop in waist measurement of 5 inches and improvements in your cholesterol and triglycerides. Or, if you are normal weight, you may not lose any more weight but still see the metabolic improvements and an increase in your energy level. If you have a history of hypoglycemia, this diet will control your insulin levels and stop your hypoglycemic episodes. The diet can be used in people who are overweight and have other diseases but in such cases, the diet must be used with your doctor's approval and with their oversight.

We hope you will give this plan a try and see for yourself.

THE AUTHORS REQUEST THAT YOU PLEASE NOTE:

With this diet or any diet or exercise program, you should consult with your personal physician before starting. He or she may need to work with you especially if you have any other medical conditions. You may be on medications (such as insulin or other blood sugar-lowering agents or water pills or blood thinners or other drugs) that can be affected by changes in diet or weight loss. Your doctor may want to screen your blood before, during, and after this diet in order to be sure it is indeed the right way for you to eat forever. This is not meant to scare you but to alert you that the diet you follow DOES have an impact on your health and well-being.

"Nothing tastes like slim feels"

Chapter One:
What You've Tried
and Why It Failed

Obesity is a major public health problem affecting the U.S. population. It is a co-factor in the outcomes of multiple diseases including cardiac disease, atherosclerosis, diabetes mellitus, and hypertension. Medical and public awareness of the problem are strong. We all know we have a serious health problem. Yet, in spite of aggressive attempts at weight loss through exercise and various calorie-reduction diets, our population taken as a whole is increasing, not decreasing, its weight. A recent survey cites that over 54% of the adult population is currently overweight as defined by a **body-mass index (BMI)** greater than 24.9 in women and men. We will explain the body-mass index later in the book. Suffice it to say that the American adults are in a state of crisis when it comes to weight and weight-related health problems.

If you just take a look around you at any large public gathering, say at church or a concert or the movies, you can readily see that we Americans have a weight problem. Normal weight people are now the minority. This is truly a sad admission. Why have we been unable to address the crisis? Clearly, we Americans will try anything when it comes to losing weight. But, sadly, even the National Institutes of Health lists its first priority in fighting this fight as trying to prevent Americans from GAINING EVEN MORE WEIGHT. Weight reduction itself is their second goal. And, they admit, it's getting harder and harder to accomplish that goal. We find sedentary lifestyles and saturated fats to be blamed. But honestly, are any of us less busy than we were 10 years ago? Sales of sports equipment are booming and early mornings find the malls loaded with walkers. Sales of "low" fat and "fat-free" items at all time highs, some reversal of this trend ought to be occurring. Obviously, just telling the public to increase exercise and eat low fat isn't the answer. What weight loss approaches have we taken to date?

Basically two non-surgical approaches have been taken towards weight loss, exercise and caloric restriction, either through restriction of total calories or calories of a specific type. Let's look at exercise first. A significant amount of exercise is needed to burn excess calories that will result in actual weight loss. This degree of effort is often not appropriate or attainable for people with severe obesity and associated diseases such as coronary artery disease or atherosclerosis. While exercise may help normal weight people maintain their weights, exercise alone is insufficient to attain weight loss in obese people. Exercise does have health benefits, however, and these benefits will be discussed in a later chapter. As a method for weight loss though, exercise can be counted on to move off a total of only 4 -7 pounds of weight, hardly a beginning for most people.

The second popular approach to weight loss has been total caloric restriction. Weight loss through severe caloric reduction (800 calories or less) has been associated with significant negative side effects, including death. The 1000-1500 calorie diets are more commonly seen and promoted by several therapeutic strategies. A review of any newsstand will reveal 1000-1500 calorie diets, promoted as "grapefruit" diets, or "cabbage" diets touted by a variety of movie and television stars, all based on the principle of caloric restriction. For-profit corporations have their own versions of the same concept complete with their own prepared foods. These calorie-restricted diets can produce weight loss, however as much as two-thirds of this weight is often regained within one year of such a diet regimen. Almost all participants regain their weight at the end of five years. Furthermore, these types of diet can result in loss of muscle mass in addition to, or in excess of, fat stores. This is not the result we want! We want weight loss to come from fat stores, the kind of weight that is around the waist and hips, not from the muscles of our biceps and triceps. Also, if a calorie-restricted diet is used, it is often necessary to take supplemental vitamins and nutrients. Failure to do so can result in nutritional deficiencies. With the liquid protein diets in particular (those diets of 800 calories or less), severe complications can occur if all supplements are not taken. Deaths have been attributed to electrolyte imbalances and loss of cardiac muscle function on these types of diets. This type of diet is very unnatural, since the components bear no relationship to normal foods. Consequently, when you go back to normal eating, the weight gain returns. Behavioral modification is often used in conjunction with these diet programs, but once again, follow-up shows failure in most cases by five years with return of the lost weight.

Surgical methods have also been tried to reduce total caloric intake. These have taken the creative forms of jaw wiring to reduce oral intake of solid, presumably high calorie foods and gastric stapling or intragastric balloons to reduce the amount of food that the stomach can hold. These major surgical procedures are often reserved for the most morbidly obese patient, precisely the type of person who is also most likely to have complications from surgery. Because of the risk of blood clots, failure to heal, and increased lung infections after surgery in obese patients, these procedures are seen less and less often.

In addition to obesity, hyperlipidememia and hypercholesterolemia (significant coronary artery disease risk factors) are increasingly prominent in the population. Taking both factors into consideration, increased weight and increased cholesterol, the use of a calorie-restricted, fat-restricted diet has been supported. Low fat diets have received widespread endorsement and promotion through such organizations as the American Dietetic Association, the American Heart Association, and the Food and Drug Administration. Individual proprietary products that meet the standards of low fat may even carry endorsements on their label such as "This product meets American Heart Association dietary guidelines for healthy people over age 2 when used as part of a balanced diet. Diets low in saturated fat and cholesterol and high in grains, fruits and vegetables that contain fiber, particularly soluble fiber, may reduce risk of heart disease, a condition associated with many factors." These types of marketing efforts have increased the demand for low fat foods. Yet, in spite of increased sales of low fat and fat-free foods, the public continues to gain weight. Are the low fat items failing or is there yet more to this picture? Clearly, low fat alone isn't the answer.

Excess carbohydrate calorie ingestion has also been implicated as a reason for weight gain. The popular press contains many titles by diet doctors attributing weight gain to uncontrolled ingestion of carbohydrates by so-called "carbohydrate addicts" or by excess carbohydrate-to-noncarbohydrate ratios in the daily diet. The central assumptions are that susceptible individuals still consume too many total calories and that these calories tend to be excess carbohydrates. Such diet authors' goals of therapy are to reduce total caloric consumption, emphasizing carbohydrate ingestion as the site for which the dieter can find these excess calories to reduce. Unfortunately, when people are not able to eat carbohydrates, they have only two other main sources of calories, fats and proteins. Excess protein can be harmful in people with kidney and liver disease. Excess fats can be harmful in up to 30% of people who are "fat-sensitive". If fat-sensitive individuals ingest any old type of fat, they may actually increase their risk of cardiac disease in the process of losing weight.

What about drug therapies? A variety of drugs have been tried to suppress appetite or to artificially increase the body's metabolic rate. Some doctors have used diuretics (so-called "water pills") to cause weight loss by dehydrating the body with the dangerous side effect of electrolyte depletion. Bulking agents containing non-digestible fiber have been given to fool the body into thinking it has eaten. Others have tried using thyroid hormone, amphetamines, and other sympathetic nervous system-stimulating drugs that have the side effect of increasing basal metabolic rate. The sympathetic nervous system puts the body in a ready state for "flight or fight". Drugs that increase sympathetic tone get the body ready for stress by increasing heart rate, blood pressure, alertness, and so forth. These processes burn more energy in the short term, but that happens so that the body can react to environmental stress. The idea behind increasing the body's own metabolic rate artificially through drugs is that more calories will be burned at rest, as if the body was in a constant state of readiness, so you can eat the same calories and lose weight. But again, dangerous problems such as sleep deprivation, drug addiction, and cardiac arrhythmias can occur. Some agents combined appetite suppressants with stimulants of metabolic rate. Such combinations have been associated with a fatal form of heart disease known as "primary pulmonary hypertension" and are currently off the market.

Another approach to weight loss has been psychological, or behavioral, modification with or without drugs. Of course, broadly speaking, whatever diet you use will involve a change in your behavior. But, what we are referring to here is the idea that there is a central defect in psychological structure that promotes abnormal eating. If that were true, then it follows that if we could restructure that pattern, the weight gain would stop. In some cases, drugs are used when it is felt that the person has characteristic features of an "obsession". While some people may suffer from obsessive behavior with regard to food, it is unlikely that this explains the national crisis. But, some behavioral modification in terms of learning new behaviors will be needed by anyone who proceeds with this or any weight loss program. That's normal and doesn't need any assistance by drug therapy.

In this section we have tried to review the major ways people have tried to lose weight. You've probably been through many of them. There's no question that it's frustrating, and frustrating to a lot of us every day. At this point, let us remind you of how bad it is. National surveys show that something like one in every three women and one in every four men are currently trying to lose weight and both sexes have spent about half of the last year on some type of diet. Help! Why are these many, many treatments failing us?

One of the fundamental reasons that weight loss keeps eluding us is that we have strayed from eating right. That is, we have been overzealous in our attraction to pre-packaged, processed foods and the content of most of these processed foods is overabundant in terms of carbohydrate, in particular sugars. Americans consume more sugar per capita than anywhere else in the world. Even our natural, unprocessed foods, like fruits, have been engineered to meet the tastes of the market, which in the U.S. calls for increasing sugar content. *Sugar consumption, both artificially added granulated sugar and corn syrup and "naturally" enhanced sugars in our foods, is one of the major problems affecting weight gain.* Now, don't say, "That doesn't apply to me. I don't eat sweets, I only eat fresh fruits." Well, sad to say, we eat TOO MANY fruits and fruit juices, too. Our fruits are not the same fruits that our ancestors ate. They only consumed fruits "in season," not year around. And their fruits were lower in sugar content than what we're eating today.

What if you say, "But I never eat sweets or fruits either." Then you need to be reminded that starches are immediately broken down into sugars by enzymes in the digestive tract so, in effect, if you're eating anything made from milled flour, pasta, rice, or potatoes, you're still getting sugars.

A second problem affecting weight gain and health concerns the high consumption of saturated fats in the diet. The average American diet consists of unhealthy amounts of saturated fat which, when combined with high carbohydrates, produces the scenario for promoting cardiac disease, hypertension, and diabetes. A future chapter will cover the mechanisms in greater detail (and there are many more things we'll share with you concerning other nutrients). But, when you look at the many, many ways we Americans have tried to lose weight, you can now see that none of these addressed completely these fundamental problems.

So, we suggest that it was not you who failed, but the methods which failed. You can do it if you have the right tools. So, let's get on with it. Ready—set—*let's "G-O."*

Chapter Two:
The Goldberg-O'Mara Diet

The last thing you want to do is to read through countless pages to get to the message. So we've decided to put down just the weight loss diet in this chapter, without commentary. You can read this section through, and then decide for yourself if this is the weight loss diet for you. Afterwards, you can read the why, how, and wherefore. If you decide not to proceed, you will save a lot of reading.

Remember, the weight loss part of this diet is meant for fatties. Later, we will tell you about our philosophy about healthy eating in general and how to modify the diet for life-long health. But here, we're dealing with the nitty-gritty, the weight loss part of the book. Some of our program may seem regimented at the beginning. That's because we know you need to get into it with both feet. You've already tried many of the things we talked about in the last chapter. They didn't work. You need this plan. So, like we said in the Introduction, give it a try for three months. If you're like our study subjects were, you'll find yourself pleasantly lighter, thinner, and healthier in three months. Then, hopefully, you'll find yourself convinced enough to continue the diet until you have achieved your final weight loss. Of course, we think that this diet could be your new way of life. So, *let's get "G-O-ing."*

Getting Started: The Body-Mass Index

This is a weight loss diet for people who have a **body mass index (BMI)** of greater than 25. The BMI is a measurement of your weight corrected for your body surface area using the formula, weight in kilograms divided by the square of your height in meters. You don't need a scientific calculator. We have included a table at the end of this chapter in which you can find your BMI. **First, find your height in feet and inches and then, locate your weight in pounds. Where the two points meet on the chart is the intersection that is your personal BMI, your starting point.** If your height falls between two points, then average the results between them.

Why not take a moment and measure your BMI? While you're at it, get out a tape measure and make a measurement of your waist at the belly button and your hips at their widest part. Write all of these measurements on a piece of paper and tuck it into a dresser drawer.

We want you to pull that paper out again in 12 weeks and make the same measurements again. Will you be surprised!

The World Health Organization has classified weight as BMI up to 25 being desirable, 25-29.9 as being overweight and 30 or greater as clinically obese. If your BMI is greater than 27, you are about 20% or more than your desirable body weight, we know you'll need this diet. If you are less than a BMI of 25, you may also try this diet. If your weight is normal, don't expect to lose weight. But you may feel better eating this way. This diet has also been shown to be useful in people with hypoglycemia, hyperinsidinemia, and insulin resistance.

The Goldberg-O'Mara Diet is a high monounsaturated fat, very low carbohydrate, nutritionally balanced diet with normal calories and normal protein levels. We repeat, normal calories! There is no counting of calories or calorie restrictions ever. We focus on only a couple of measurements, mainly carbohydrates and saturated fat and fiber.

"Very low carbohydrate" in our diet means that your carbohydrate goal will be a total daily intake of 50 grams of NET carbohydrate with not more than 12-15 grams of NET carbohydrate taken at any single meal. Carbohydrates are sugars and starches, the kinds of substances in potatoes, rice, pasta, cookies, cakes, bagels, and bread. In general, these will be excluded foods. But, you'll learn about eating an excellent diet without having high sugar and starch foods.

"High monounsaturated fat" means that 50% or more of your dietary fat will be in the form of monounsaturated fats. You already know from our previous chapter that you should keep saturated fats as low as possible. (We will also encourage some omega 3 and 6 fatty acids and polyunsaturated fats, although not in cooking. More about that later). Examples of foods that are high in monounsaturated fats include most nuts, edible seeds, canola and olive oil, olives, and avocados. But many meats, such as lean chicken and beef, already have close to 50% of their fats as monounsaturated.

"Nutritionally-balanced" means that the diet will also promote natural sources of vitamins, fiber, and other nutrients that are essential for good health. Whatever diet you follow should encourage the use of foods that provide essential vitamins and minerals. The use of fiber, antioxidants, and phytochemicals obtained from natural sources has been associated with risk reduction from some types of cancer and other diseases. The carbohydrate content from fiber is NOT limited in the **Goldberg-O'Mara Diet.** We'd like to see these substances as part of a healthy eating program.

We would like to transition you to the **Goldberg-O'Mara Diet** in three phases. First, you must abruptly cut the carbohydrates in your diet. Second, we'll work on developing the high monounsaturated fats in your diet. Finally, we will balance the nutrients from natural sources. Are you motivated? Then, read on.

What are carbohydrates?

Carbohydrates are starches and sugars. These are the substances that are driving your weight gain, your overeating, and snacking. If you will indulge us a little, we bet that we could guess your eating habits. How about this? Bagel or cereal, coffee, and juice for breakfast, followed by a "little piece" of coffee cake and coffee at 10:00 break time, followed by a burger, fries, and a cola around noon, followed by a candy bar or cookies and coffee at about 2:00. Then there's the snack of chips or pretzels and pop in the car or on the train, followed by a couple of chips or cookies while making dinner which will include pasta, potato, or rice as a side dish. A little dessert and maybe a cookie before bed? With a few variations (maybe soup and salad with bread at lunch), we'd bet this is pretty close to what you're eating when you're not on a grapefruit or cabbage diet! We need to start our diet by stopping this pattern of eating excessive amounts of carbohydrates immediately.

How to Count Carbohydrates

You will need to count the carbohydrate content of all foods that you eat. Carbohydrate amounts of common sized portions of many foods can be found in nutrition books, carbohydrate counters, and on the nutrition labels of processed foods. Buy a pocket-sized carbohydrate counter to have with you at all times during the first couple of weeks on the diet until you are accustomed to the content in common foods. See our chart in **Appendix 1** to get you started immediately.

You are interested in the "net" carbohydrates. This is calculated by subtracting the amount of fiber from the total carbohydrate count. FIBER DOESN'T COUNT. Since we hinted to you earlier that fiber has some beneficial properties, you can guess what's coming. You can eat as much fiber as you want! And we want you to aim for a goal of at least 25 grams of fiber daily. So, remember this formula:

Net Carbohydrates = Total Carbohydrates - Fiber

You only restrict your NET CARBOHYDRATES.

During the first three days of the transition to the Goldberg-O'Mara way of eating, we want you to concentrate solely on the net carbohydrate count of the foods you eat. This is probably the hardest part of the diet. But, we know you're motivated, so let's move to that first phase now.

Phase One: Your first three days

In Transition on the Goldberg-O'Mara Diet

Let's put you on a strict diet for the first three days. This will give your body a chance to gear up for burning fat. The little furnaces in your cells called mitochondria are where the fat is burned. We need to send a loud and clear message to those fat burning machines that they are going to increase production. All leave has been canceled and they are going to be putting in a lot of overtime. And it will give you a chance to shop and change from the fat-free, high carbohydrate household you've been living in into one in which you can lose some serious weight.

Eat as much as you like (within the 12- 15 gram NET carbohydrate per meal and 50 gram NET carbohydrate per day limit) of the foods on the table called **"The Goldberg-O'Mara Diet First Three Days"**. DON'T EAT ANYTHING THAT IS NOT ON THIS TABLE. NOT EVEN A TASTE. We mean that very strongly. If you want this diet to work for you, then start out with this three day regimen. The later **"Science and the Diet"** chapter will explain why and it will make sense.

Broil, bake, grill, boil, pan-fry. If pan-frying, cook all foods in olive or canola oil. Use oil-and-vinegar or unsweetened, full fat salad dressings. READ ALL PACKAGE LABELS for carbohydrate content. Drink diet pop, coffee, tea, water, plain or artificially sweetened kefir, or buttermilk. No other milk of any type is allowed. Please refrain from any alcohol for these first three days.

Eat three meals a day and snack whenever you feel like it. DON'T SKIP ANY MEALS. Use cheese cubes, string cheese, tuna , chicken drumsticks or wings (roasted, seasoned with salt-and-pepper, dipped in no-carbohydrate condiments) for snacks.

Because you're just starting, and *this is a Transition Phase Diet*, take one multivitamin-and-mineral supplement a day. Also, don't count calories. We mean it sincerely, DO NOT COUNT CALORIES OR FAT DURING THESE FIRST THREE DAYS. You are concentrating on one goal during the first three days. That goal is getting the carbohydrates out of your eating pattern.

The Goldberg-O'Mara Diet: First Three Days

Meats/Fish/Nuts	*Dairy*	*Vegetables*
Any meat, trimmed of all excess fat and unbreaded	Kefir, Yogurt or buttermilk, plain, unsweetened or sweetened by you with artificial sweeteners.	Cucumbers, lettuce, greens, spinach, olives, broccoli, cauliflower, mushrooms, celery, Chinese vegetables, zucchini, onions, asparagus, squash
Any fish or shellfish, unbreaded		
Canned fish in oil	Cheeses, unsweetened:	
All nuts, except pistachios and cashews	Cheddar, Swiss, Mozarella, Ricotta, Cream, Cottage	**Other:**
Edible seeds (sunflower kernels, pumpkin seeds)	Real cream	Eggs, mayonnaise, sugar -free condiments Sour pickles.

Sugar free gelatin, spices, salt, pepper, no-calorie sweeteners

Sample "First Three Days" menus
(Note that the amounts of these foods are not limited except for the 12-15 gram NET carbohydrate per meal and 50 gram net carbohydrate per day limit.)

Breakfast Suggestions
• Plain kefir drink-with nuts and sunflower kernels on the side

• Plain yogurt-mixed with nuts, cinnamon, no-calorie sweetener to taste

• Ham and cheese omelet

- Scrambled eggs and breakfast sausage

- Nuts and cheese cubes or string cheese

Lunch Suggestions
- Chef's salad: mixed greens, turkey, cheese, ham, hard-boiled egg

- Cheeseburgers without the bun, side salad, no carbohydrate condiments

- Tuna on a bed of lettuce with hard-boiled eggs

- Stir fried vegetables in oil and chicken breast

- Cheese-stuffed portobello mushrooms and salad

- Assorted cold cuts and cucumber salad with sour cream

Dinner Suggestions
- Grilled lean steak, large spinach salad, stir-fried zucchini

- Roast chicken, mashed cauliflower, broccoli with cheese, salad

- Baked whitefish, asparagus, stir-fried mushrooms, mixed greens salad

- Stir fried lean beef and Chinese vegetables (no rice)

Desserts and Snacks
- Sugar-free, flavored gelatin and whipped cream

- Flavored coffees (no syrups), no-calorie sweeteners, and cream

- Cheese cubes and nuts

- Ricotta cheese and cinnamon, no-calorie sweetener

- Hard-boiled eggs

- Chicken drumsticks and wings

- Kefir or yogurt shake, use no-calorie sweeteners

Maybe you are thinking, how can I live without my potatoes, rice, pasta or bread? We urge you to try some of the great foods we've just outlined. There is no question that some of you will find these first three days very hard. Why that occurs will be explained in the next chapter. But remember, don't give in to the temptation to cheat. NOT EVEN A TASTE OF ANYTHING THAT'S NOT ON THIS LIST. You need these three days of strict control to get you started. It will get easier. Be sure to have canned tuna, cheese cubes, hard-boiled eggs, and chicken wings around in case you get "shaky".

Next, we go to...

Phase Two: Promoting High Monounsaturated Fats

Transitioning Days 4-7

Now you have the idea of living on very low carbohydrates. Your intake has been so low that you are starting to burn fat. Now we have to work on the kinds of fats you are eating so that your diet will be safe for you over the long haul. During phase two, after your first three days, we will work on promoting those foods that contain high monounsaturated fats to shift the balance away from saturated fats in your diet.

Saturated fats, those fats associated with promoting heart disease., are solids at room temperature. We can have some of these fats, probably 40 grams or less a day. Since fats are a large component of your new diet, it is critical to be eating the right kinds of fats, *high monounsaturated fats.* You have completed your first three days and you should now take the time to look ahead to the section on shopping so that you can have more variety in your diet.

How do you make the diet high in monounsaturated fats? One goal of the diet is to maintain your fat intake composition to at least 50% monounsaturated fatty acids (MUFAs). This may sound complicated, but it is really very easy. **Appendix 1** lists allowable foods with their carbohydrate counts and their percentage of monounsaturated fats. As you will notice, most meats, fish, and chicken already contain over 40% MUFAs. So supplementation of your diet with a few foods containing very high levels of MUFAs will easily bring you over the 50% level. Dairy products on the other hand have less than 30% MUFAs. So if you eat a lot of cheese, you will have to eat a lot more of the high-MUFA foods such as canola oil, olive oil, nuts, and avocados.

Examples to increase percentage of MUFAs:
- A meal of steak and a salad with olive oil and vinegar dressing will have over 50% MUFA.

- Increase MUFA in a kefir shake by adding 1 tbsp. of canola oil

- A meal of a two-egg omelet with cheddar cheese is acceptable provided you fry it in olive oil

- Snacking on nuts and seeds and eating less meat helps your daily totals

Many of us had given up nuts thinking that they put weight on because of their high fat content. Not so! Nuts and seeds are excellent sources of the RIGHT FATS, monounsaturated fats, and fiber. So, rediscover nuts and edible seeds. Ground-up nuts can be used to make pie crusts. Chopped nuts and seeds in yogurt and on all-bran, high fiber cereals taste great.

Avocados are also high in monounsaturated fats. Guacamole and other avocado salads are great tasting high MUFA foods that can improve your MUFA intake. Try a chicken taco salad with extra guacamole.

So don't get into a panic about your 50% MUFA target. Remember to have canola and olive oils, nuts and seeds, and olives and avocados readily available in your kitchen. Just get into the habit of dressing salads with olive oil, stir-frying veggies and meats with oil, tossing oil into vegetables instead of butter, eating avocados and snacking on nuts and seeds. And, as always, trim meats of excess fat, and skim soups and stews of any fats that you can see on top.

Phase Three: Making the Diet Nutritionally Sound
End of Week One- Lifetime of healthy eating

By this time, you are well into the diet. You have passed your first three days on the strict carbohydrate clearance. You have moved into increasing your selection of foods by adding extra monounsaturated fats. More nuts and seeds, less fatty meats and sausages. More fish and grilled meats, less high saturated fat-prepared meats. Oil dressings over Russian or French. You are an expert in these areas and you have probably been eating on the diet plan for about a week now. You have seen some weight loss. Now let's refine the diet plan even further and make it complete, something you can live with for the long haul safely.

We hope you have jumped ahead to read the chapter on shopping and that your pantry is cleared of those high carbohydrate rice cakes, pretzels, and bagels. We're willing to bet there were plenty there. The "Nutrition Facts" labels on the processed foods in your old pantry probably startled you. Can you believe the amount of carbohydrates you were eating?

Hopefully, you have started to look at the **"Recipes"** section for some new ideas. You now know how to increase your dietary intake of high monounsaturated fats. What else do we need to consider? *Increasing fiber, adding fermented milk products, adding natural sources of vitamins and minerals.*

High Fiber

Your diet needs high fiber, both soluble and insoluble. Fiber has a beneficial effect upon cholesterol by binding it and preventing its reabsorption. It is a natural laxative and it may have a role in the protection against some cancers. How do we increase fiber in the diet? We do this by increasing our consumption of bran, the husk part of grains. You have to go back to the store in order to find wheat, oat, and corn brans. Search for these in the section of the store that sells flours and dry, bulk items. Or look for them at your health food store. Don't give up! Wheat bran is usually the easiest to find. Oat bran has the highest net carbohydrates but its flavor is tastier. You may have no luck in finding corm bran but it is probably tastiest of all.

DON'T confuse labels stating "whole wheat" or "wheat germ" as being equivalent to wheat bran. They're not. There's little or no fiber in those items. Likewise, don't think that "natural oats" or "bran cereal" contain any meaningful fiber. They cannot substitute for wheat or oat brans. Make sure you're buying the right stuff.

You can use wheat bran to make pancakes or waffles. Use wheat bran as a breading for fried fish and chicken. You can use it as a "filler" when making meatballs or meatloaf. You can mix wheat and oat brans together and cook with water to create your own hot cereal. Again, as you are experimenting, do that math. Make sure your final product will still have a low NET carbohydrate count and will fit into your meal allowance.

Ground flax seeds are a also wonderful source of soluble and insoluble fiber and are loaded with omega-3 and 6 fatty acids and so-called "phytoestrogens". These versatile tiny brown seeds when ground, can make a substitute hot cereal when you add boiling water. Flaxseed has a slightly bitter aftertaste so you may want to add cinnamon to your cereal. Adding flaxseed to oat bran will increase the nutrients while preserving the oat bran taste.

Another way to increase fiber is through high fiber-containing vegetables. Some examples of high fiber vegetables are avocados, bamboo shoots, broccoli, brussel sprouts, cauliflower, cabbage, green beans and spinach. Nuts and seeds are also good sources of fiber.

Psyllium husks are considered a natural laxative because of their soluble fiber content. You can use psyllium husks in cooking as a thickening agent for gravies where you would have previously used white flour or cornstarch. Psyllium is also an excellent binder for meatballs and meatloaf where you previously would have used breadcrumbs or cereal. If you need to hide it to get it in, try sugar-free, flavored psyllium products stirred into club soda. It can also be added as 1 teaspoon to plain yogurt or kefir in a breakfast shake.

Check the fiber contents of foods to maximize the amount of fiber you take in daily. There are some premade cereals that are extra high in fiber and are suitable for this diet. One popular cereal manufacturer has a high fiber cereal with 13 grams of fiber per 1/2 cup serving. Combine 1/2 cup of this cereal with 1oz. of sunflower kernels, 1 oz. of walnuts, a little no-calorie sweetener and some whole cream or kefir and you will have an excellent breakfast with over 20 grams of fiber and under 15 grams of net carbohydrates. **Try to aim for 25 grams or more of fiber a day**. It will be a challenge at first because you're not accustomed to thinking about these high fiber foods. But it's important for your health. And by now, you are starting to feel the benefits of your healthier eating.

Keep reading for more nutritional additions to the diet.

Fermented Milk Products

There has been a lot of press in the recent years about yeast overgrowth and its effects on your health and well being. There is some reason to believe that high carbohydrate diets and the overuse of some drugs, like antibiotics, may promote abnormal yeast overgrowth in and on the body. One natural way to combat this problem is to use an ancient remedy that is natural and well tolerated by anyone. This remedy is to restore healthy bacteria to your body in the form of cultured milk products such as kefir, yogurt, and buttermilk.

A bacterium called "lactobacillus" is a very important conditioner of the human gastrointestinal tract. You can take pills, but again, we feel it is better to use natural sources. It is much more delicious to take your bacteria in live culture kefir, yogurt, or buttermilk. Any of these three products can, and SHOULD, be used as part of your daily diet. Of the three choices, kefir may have even additional benefits because of the other "good" microorganisms it contains. Kefir is made from cultures containing a specific mixture of bacteria and "friendly" yeasts that are obtained from the kefir grain. There are currently research projects being undertaken in the United States to assess whether there are additional benefits to kefir. There are patents on anticancer substances extracted from kefir grains. This product has been widely used in western Europe, having originated several centuries ago.

Recent research has shown that among its many good qualities, these bacteria also stimulate the body to produce important immune response chemicals called "cytokines". These molecules include interferons and tumor necrosis factor and therefore might improve our resistance to disease. They also form a great deal of bulk for the formation of well-formed, non-constipating stools. Even lactose-intolerant individuals can tolerate kefir, yogurt and buttermilk. That is because the lactose in the milk used to make these products has been digested by the "good" lactobacillus. For example, the actual lactose left in kefir made by a national manufacturer is 1% or less. IN THIS CASE ONLY, AND WITH THESE FOODS ONLY, don't count the carbohydrate on the package labels. Why not?

The problem with the stated carbohydrate content on the packages of fermented food products arises because the government makes manufacturers count the carbohydrates of food "by difference". That means they measure everything else including water and ash and fats and proteins. Then "by difference," they assume everything else is carbohydrate. This works quite well for most foods including milk. However, to make yogurt, buttermilk and kefir, the milk is inoculated with the lactic acid bacteria. These bacteria use up almost all the milk sugar called "lactose" and convert it into lactic acid. It is this lactic acid which curds the milk and gives the taste to the product. Since these bacteria have "eaten" most of the milk sugar by the time you buy it or if you make it yourself. At the time you eat it, how can there be much carbohydrate left?

It is the lactic acid which is counted as carbohydrate. Therefore, you can eat up to a half cup of plain yogurt, buttermilk, or kefir and only count 2 grams of carbohydrates (Dr. Goldberg has measured this in his own laboratory). One cup will contain about 4 grams of carbohydrates. Daily consumption colonizes the intestine with these bacteria to handle small amounts of lactose in yogurt (or even sugar-free ice cream later). Look ahead to the recipe chapter on making your own delicious yogurts and kefirs.

When you go to buy ready-made kefir and yogurt, look for plain, unsweetened or artificially sweetened varieties. Don't be afraid of plain, unsweetened varieties. This is how kefir and yogurt have traditionally been used. So many cultures have used these products that when you tell your grandmother about your new diet, she may inform you it's not new at all. She may share her yogurt or kefir making stories from her childhood. You may find that "plain" tastes best of all when you come to appreciate the historical significance. Or, you can be trendy and add your own no-calorie sweeteners and flavorings (or berries or nuts and seeds).

It may be better if the product is "bovine growth hormone free" although this is still controversial. Does it matter if it's "nonfat", "low fat" or "original, normal fat"? No. This will affect the texture a bit, but on this diet, you can eat any fat content product. Your preference rules here. We prefer the "mouth feel" of the whole milk varieties. But, try them all and decide for yourself. You should also get a little gutsy now and try cheeses made from kefir and yogurt. These products are available ready made or you can make them yourself. Again, your grandmother may have the best technique or you can see our recipes at the end. **Aim for at least 8 ounces of kefir, yogurt, or buttermilk daily.**

Another point about adding fermented milk products. Remember that milk products made from milk that has been supplemented with calcium becomes an important source of calcium in the diet. Since this diet does not allow you to drink regular milk, it is very important to include vitamin D and calcium-supplemented fermented milk products for their calcium content as well as the other beneficial effects that we cited above.

Natural Sources of Vitamins and Minerals

A great, healthy diet needs a little more to round it out. We need to pay attention to natural sources of vitamins and minerals. **Your diet should contain <u>at least</u> five servings of assorted vegetables daily.** These vegetables should represent a variety of dark green, leafy, and yellow vegetables to provide natural sources of many vitamins and minerals. Nuts and edible seeds are imperative and will provide potassium, magnesium, vitamin E and other antioxidants. High fiber, low sugar content fruits such as kiwi, berries, rhubarb, and melon can be included up to 1/2 cup daily.

Grains and cereals that are very high in fiber, and therefore proportionally low in net carbohydrates, should be part of the diet. Such grains include flaxseed, wheat bran, oat bran, and corn bran. Flaxseed has an additional benefit of containing high omega 3 and 6 fatty acids and natural antioxidants. It is felt to be beneficial against some types of cancer. Read labels very carefully if buying processed foods. Wherever possible, unprocessed forms of foods should be used.

As you have read this chapter and built your new diet, you have moved to a healthy way of eating. You've gone from a weight loss plan to a diet plan that may promote good health over a lifetime. Your diet now has reduced net carbohydrates, enhanced monoun-saturated fats, reduced saturated fats, increased fiber, increased natural sources of vitamins, minerals, and antioxidants, increased fermented milk products with normal calorie and protein levels. And, you'll lose excess weight on it. Let's review the final diet on the next two pages.

Summary of Foods Allowed on the Goldberg-O'Mara Diet

MEATS
(Try to substitute low saturated fat choices and have non-meat lunches and dinners)

Lean, non-breaded beef, chicken, turkey, lamb, veal, pork, all-meat sausages and hot dogs, luncheon meats

FISH
(Look for ways to increase intake)

Non-breaded fish and shellfish Canned fish packed in oil or water

CHEESE/DAIRY/EGGS
(Push those underlined into your daily diet)

All cheeses (check carbohydrate content if processed); heavy cream, yogurt, kefir, buttermilk, sour cream; eggs

VEGETABLES
(5 or more servings a day)

All , except for the following: NO potatoes, sweet potatoes, rice, peas, beans and lentils (green, pole, and wax beans are okay)

NUTS/SEEDS

Spanish peanuts, pecans, walnuts, hazelnuts, almonds, macadamia nuts, edible seeds

FRUITS

Up to 1/2 cup of berries, rhubarb, melon, kiwi fruit. Up to 1/2 of a small low-sugar, tart apple or pear

BEVERAGES

tea, coffee, diet sodas, diet tonic water, club soda, plain kefir, no-calorie powdered drink mixes; alcohol to be limited to 1 mixed drink or 1 light beer or 5 oz. dry red or white wine/day

Summary of Foods Allowed *continued*

DESSERTS

artificially sweetened gelatin, egg-based custards, mousses, dessert cheeses, berries and cream, yogurt or kefir smoothies and shakes

HIGH FIBER FOODS
(Strongly encouraged-25 grams daily)

wheat, corn and oat bran, flaxseed, psyllium husks, nuts, seeds, many vegetables

CONDIMENTS

Oil and vinegar, mustard, mayonnaise, pickles, olives, peppers, spices, iodized salt, pepper, butter, sugar free sauces.

A Few More Things About Using the Diet

Excluded Foods
There are some foods you will just have to forget about because they are so high in carbohydrates that even a small portion is a signifi-cant load. **So, here's the list of the no-nos:** NO milk, potatoes, sweet potatoes, beets, turnips, rice, corn, peas, beans (except green, wax, pole), lentils, pasta, breads, bagels, cookies, cakes, most crackers, pretzels, rice cakes.

Helpful Suggestions
Get involved. Planning of menus and careful shopping are impor-tant. If you have your supplies on hand you will be less tempted to break the diet. If you want to eat out, stick to the following rules:

• Never order the soup unless its beef, chicken, or vegetable consommé. No noodles, croutons or crackers.

• No breads or pasta or potatoes or rice. If you order a burger, throw away the bun or ask for extra pickles or lettuce as a substitute. Ask for salad substitute or other vegetables or tomato slices instead of the potato or pasta side. Don't let the waitress even leave bread or crackers at the table.

- Make your own salad dressing from oil and vinegar.

- Scrape off any breading and leave it on your bread plate.

- Ask for cheese and strawberries or strawberries and cream for dessert. You can sweeten it with the no-calorie sweetener on the table if you need to.

- Ask Chinese restaurants not to thicken your sauce with starch or flour. Better to have foods simply stir-fried without sauces.

- Remember that you can eat meat, chicken, fish or eggs without any portion controls. But, pile on the low carbohydrate veggies and salads at every opportunity. Order extra sides of vegetables. And always trim excess fat.

Good luck. Don't get angry with yourself if you fall off the wagon and cheat. Old habits will be hard to break. Just look yourself in the mirror and say the following to your image. Say it in a loud voice so you can hear it, "Are you serious about losing weight? Then I don't want this to happen again. You are not a child. Grow up and take responsibility for yourself. There was no reason to eat that unhealthy junk."

Then get right back on the diet at the point you left off. You don't have to go through the first phase again. You still have your fat burning enzymes. It will take your body two or three days to recover from the carbohydrate shock, but then you'll be back in the saddle again. However, if you break the diet for more than two meals, you will have to start at square one again. Later, when you have lost most of your weight, you will find the same holds true for diet vacations. For example, if you visit a country that is famous for a particular dish, try it once, then get right back on the diet. Your body will always forgive these little indiscretions so long as you remain in control. If ever you feel you are losing control, IMMEDI-ATELY RETURN TO THE PHASE ONE TRANSITION DIET.

OK. That's the diet. Now onto the science.

Table 1. Find Your BMI

If your height fall between two numbers, estimate your BMI by averaging.

Your Weight in Pounds	4'10"	5'0"	5'2"	5'4"	5'6"	5'8"	5'10"	6'0"	6'2"	6'4"	6'6"	6'8"
95	19.9	18.6	17.4	16.4	15.4	14.5						
100	21.0	19.6	18.4	17.2	16.2	15.3	14.4					
105	22.0	20.6	19.3	18.1	17.0	16.0	15.1	14.3				
110	23.1	21.6	20.2	18.9	17.8	16.8	15.8	15.0	14.2			
115	24.1	22.5	21.1	19.8	18.6	17.5	16.6	15.7	14.8	14.0		
120	25.2	23.5	22.0	20.7	19.4	18.3	17.3	16.3	15.5	14.7		
125	26.2	24.5	22.9	21.5	20.2	19.1	18.0	17.0	16.1	15.3	14.5	
130	27.3	25.5	23.9	22.4	21.1	19.8	18.7	17.7	16.8	15.9	15.1	14.3
135	28.3	26.5	24.8	23.3	21.9	20.6	19.4	18.4	17.4	16.5	15.7	14.9
140	29.4	27.4	25.7	24.1	22.7	21.4	20.2	19.1	18.0	17.1	16.2	15.4
145	30.4	28.4	26.6	25.0	23.5	22.1	20.9	19.7	18.7	17.7	16.8	16.0
150	31.5	29.4	27.5	25.8	24.3	22.9	21.6	20.4	19.3	18.3	17.4	16.5
155	32.5	30.4	28.5	26.7	25.1	23.7	22.3	21.1	20.0	18.9	18.0	17.1
160	33.6	31.4	29.4	27.6	25.9	24.4	23.0	21.8	20.6	19.5	18.6	17.6
165	34.6	32.3	30.3	28.4	26.7	25.2	23.8	22.5	21.3	20.2	19.1	18.2
170	35.7	33.3	31.2	29.3	27.5	25.9	24.5	23.1	21.9	20.8	19.7	18.7
175	36.7	34.3	32.1	30.1	28.3	26.7	25.2	23.8	22.5	21.4	20.3	19.3
180	37.8	35.3	33.0	31.0	29.2	27.5	25.9	24.5	23.2	22.0	20.9	19.8
185	38.8	36.3	34.0	31.9	30.0	28.2	26.6	25.2	23.8	22.6	21.5	20.4
190	39.9	37.2	34.9	32.7	30.8	29.0	27.4	25.9	24.5	23.2	22.0	20.9
195	40.9	38.2	35.8	33.6	31.6	29.8	28.1	26.5	25.1	23.8	22.6	21.5
200	42.0	39.2	36.7	34.5	32.4	30.5	28.8	27.2	25.8	24.4	23.2	22.1
205	43.0	40.2	37.6	35.3	33.2	31.3	29.5	27.9	26.4	25.0	23.8	22.6
210	44.0	41.2	38.5	36.2	34.0	32.0	30.2	28.6	27.1	25.7	24.4	23.2
215	45.1	42.1	39.5	37.0	34.8	32.8	31.0	29.3	27.7	26.3	24.9	23.7
220	46.1	43.1	40.4	37.9	35.6	33.6	31.7	29.9	28.3	26.9	25.5	24.3
225	47.2	44.1	41.3	38.8	36.4	34.3	32.4	30.6	29.0	27.5	26.1	24.8
230	48.2	45.1	42.2	39.6	37.3	35.1	33.1	31.3	29.6	28.1	26.7	25.4
235	49.3	46.1	43.1	40.5	38.1	35.9	33.8	32.0	30.3	28.7	27.3	25.9
240	50.3	47.0	44.1	41.3	38.9	36.6	34.6	32.7	30.9	29.3	27.8	26.5
245	51.4	48.0	45.0	42.2	39.7	37.4	35.3	33.3	31.6	29.9	28.4	27.0
250	52.4	49.0	45.9	43.1	40.5	38.1	36.0	34.0	32.2	30.5	29.0	27.6
255	53.5	50.0	46.8	43.9	41.3	38.9	36.7	34.7	32.9	31.2	29.6	28.1
260	54.5	51.0	47.7	44.8	42.1	39.7	37.4	35.4	33.5	31.8	30.2	28.7
265	55.6	51.9	48.6	45.7	42.9	40.4	38.2	36.1	34.1	32.4	30.7	29.2

Chapter Three:
Results of the Diet Study

The scientific study of any diet is of prime importance. We were the co-investigators of a research program testing the **Goldberg-O'Mara** Diet in moderate-to-severely obese subjects. This research project was conducted at a major Chicago hospital and approved by its Institutional Review Board, the committee that monitors research on human subjects.

We asked thirty volunteers to participate in the formal study of the diet. To qualify as a subject, they had to be obese, with a BMI greater than 29, have a normal thyroid gland function and not be under a physician's care for treatment of diabetes or other serious medical condition for which they were on medication. Several subjects who were hypertensive (high blood pressure) joined the study with their doctor's written permission.

After an open meeting to describe the diet and sign up the participants, each was told to eat their usual excess of carbohydrates for three days, then come to the laboratory for a fasting five-hour glucose tolerance test. If you have never undergone a glucose tolerance test, let us describe what the subjects went through. They showed up for an eight o'clock in the morning appointment, having had nothing to eat since seven o'clock on the previous evening. The laboratory phlebotomist (that's the name given to the technician who draws your blood) checked on the paperwork, measured the subject's height and weight then drew two tubes of blood from the arm. Fat people usually don't like to get their blood drawn because there is often so much fat covering the veins, the technician can have a difficult time finding the vein from which to draw the blood. However, a well trained and experienced phlebotomist can usually make this a relatively painless procedure. Those blood samples were obtained to screen the subjects for fasting blood sugar in addition to the thyroid tests and a host of other tests which checked for abnormalities of liver and kidney function, blood lipids and other markers of nutritional status.

Then we started the glucose tolerance test. Each subject was given a flavored glucose drink containing 75 grams of carbohydrate, to be completely consumed in 10 minutes. From that point on, the subjects stayed calm and remained sitting in the reception area without smoking, eating or drinking. Each hour on the hour, for the next five hours, another tube of blood was drawn. The first two hours of this test are OK. If you have a normal metabolism, the whole test is without incident. However, obese people do not have a normal metabolism and we found certain things started to happen around three to four hours into the test. Some felt nauseated; others got chills, sweats or palpitations. In any case, most of our obese subjects did not feel well. By five hours, however, everything was back to normal for most subjects and after the last tube of blood was drawn, they rushed down to the cafeteria for a late combo breakfast, lunch and snack.

Meanwhile, the blood tubes were sent to the laboratory for analysis. Each of the glucose tolerance blood samples was analyzed for both glucose and the hormone called insulin.

Once the entire battery of tests was completed and the results reviewed by us, subjects were asked to start the diet. They were told to maintain a detailed diary of their food intake and to return each week for a weigh-in and nutritional counseling.

Initial Lab Results

It was no surprise to us that 75% of subjects had a high fasting insulin when compared to the fasting insulin of people with a BMI of less than 25. (For those who are interested, the method of analysis was by the Abbott Diagnostics IMx analyzer and a "normal" result was less than 40 pmol/L). However, almost 90% had very high insulin levels at 1 and 2 hours after drinking the glucose solution (greater than 50 mU/L or greater than 360 pmol/L). Most fat people are insulin resistant. In order to keep their blood sugars normal, they must put out much more insulin than a normal weight person. The reason for this massive insulin output is resistance to the action of insulin by the muscle cells. This will be discussed further in the next chapter. But bear in mind that this is the typical response we see in Type 2 diabetics. As we will show you, diabetes and obesity are kissing cousins.

Other test results were unremarkable. Most subjects has cholesterol values in the "desirable" range (less than 200 mg/dL) and high normal triglycerides (less than 200 mg/dL) with a few exceptions. One subject had triglycerides over 800 mg/dL. A few had mild elevations in the serum enzymes that are derived from the liver. None had high uric acid, an indicator of gout and everyone had normal kidney function test results.

Into the Diet

At the weekly session, subjects were weighed and their diet diary was reviewed. If we felt they needed to modify their intake, we suggested different food choices. Interestingly, one of the main problems we found at the beginning of the diet was that subjects did not eat enough. We told you about this phenomenon before. People want to lose weight badly and often they will try to starve themselves or skip meals in order to accomplish some weight loss. THIS DIET DOESN'T WORK THAT WAY. They were so used to trying low calorie diets, they were afraid to eat. However, we quickly reassured them and made sure they had adequate food intake to prevent their bodies from slowing their metabolism because of inadequate calories. Our usual caloric intake was about 2000-2200 calories.

Another common finding was lack of fiber in the diet, which led to constipation. We emphasized that after the transition time, they had to eat at least five servings a day of vegetables and reinforced the idea eating of fermented milk products such as kefir, buttermilk or yogurt daily. This was new to most of the subjects. They were not accustomed to eating that many vegetables and that large of a variety and were unaccustomed to fermented milk products. We probably shouldn't have been surprised after describing the usual eating habits of Americans in an earlier chapter. But again, there seems to be so much stress on eating high carbohydrate cereals, pasta, and breads in the current culture, veggies have gotten lost.

It was interesting to note that many of our subjects did not cook at home. They ate most or all of their meals in the hospital cafeteria or at restaurants. This created a problem for supplementation of the diet with wheat bran and other fiber. We suggested that they eat a one hundred percent wheat bran cereal with artificially sweetened kefir for breakfast, counting the net carbohydrates to keep within the 12 -15 gram net carbohydrate per meal allowance.

Psyllium husk fiber is an excellent dietary supplement to prevent constipation and to lower cholesterol. Most people don't like to drink the commercial products. However, we suggested that the fiber could be added to pancakes, meatballs or even protein shakes for breakfast.

Our diet called for eating lots of nuts and seeds to enhance the intake of monounsaturated fats. This was well accepted by the group. They generally liked nuts and edible seeds, but had been avoiding them because of a misconception regarding their high fat content. But nuts have the good fats. Once this was understood, nuts became a mainstay dietary addition. This had a side benefit of preventing the potassium and magnesium imbalances that are common with other low carbohydrate diets. One of the symptoms of a electrolyte imbalance is severe night cramps in the calf muscles. None of our subjects experienced this problem.

Three of our subjects did not return for the first weigh-in and did not return our calls. Maybe they just wanted all the free lab work. Maybe they couldn't get through the transition phase. We don't know. During the remainder of the study we lost three more participants. One got sick and her physician insisted she stop the diet, one got severe diarrhea and thought it was due to the diet and the third couldn't give up the beer and dropped out after 3 weeks.

That left 24 participants who completed the entire 12 weeks of the study. That's an 80% compliance rate. As you read in chapter one, most dieters give up on their diets. Why then did 80% of participants stick with this diet? Is it because the diet works with no feelings of deprivation? Perhaps it is because the weight came off so easily together with an overall feeling of well-being. Whatever the reasons, a diet that retains 80% of its subjects has to be doing something right.

Ketones

Why is there a feeling of well-being? This is a difficult question to answer with facts, but initially it may have to do with the ketogenic state of a low carbohydrate intake. When the body reaches a state of carbohydrate depletion it starts to burn fat for fuel. This happens when you fast, perform long strenuous exercise or in some abnormal situations, such as Type 1 diabetes, when there is no available insulin to force the sugars into the cells.

Burning fatty acids for energy is a normal function of cells. It occurs in little power factories within the cells called "mitochondria". The fatty acids, which contain long chains of carbon atoms, are chopped up two carbon atoms at a time in a process call beta-oxidation. For example, an 18 carbon chain fatty acid will be broken down into 9 two- carbon pieces which get attached to a molecule called Coenzyme A. These pieces known as acetyl-coenzyme A (Acetyl-CoA for short), are the primary building blocks for new fatty acids and cholesterol synthesis. Most of it, however, gets burned up in the major energy producing cycle called the tricarboxylic acid or citric acid or Krebs cycle. This is the usual way that we derive energy from both carbohydrates and fats and proteins.

Under normal feeding conditions, when there are plenty of carbohydrates around, almost all of the Acetyl-CoA will go through the citric acid cycle and end up as carbon dioxide, water and energy. In times of carbohydrate starvation, when fats are being chopped up for energy, there is an excess of the Acetyl-CoA which gets shunted off into an alternative pathway in the mitochondria and ends up as compounds called "ketone bodies" and carbon dioxide.

There are two main ketone bodies produced. One is called "acetoacetic acid" and the other is named "beta-hydroxybutyric acid" (HBA). Acetoacetic acid can spontaneously break down to form acetone and this is the compound which gives people on this diet a faint, but distinct smell on their breath. Other low carbohydrate diets advocate the use of ketosticks to detect these ketones in the urine, as a sign that you are really burning fats. However, these sticks, which are expensive, only detect the acetoacetic acid and acetone, which are less than one fifth of the ketones produced. The HBA goes totally undetected by this test. Many people never produce enough acetoacetic acid to cause these sticks to turn color, yet testing their blood for HBA shows plenty of ketones.

We would therefore suggest that you ignore the use of ketosticks. It may be interesting for you to use it as a check for ketosis, but it has nothing to do with your rate of weight loss. We have seen people positive for urine ketones who don't lose weight, and people who are negative for ketones rapidly losing weight. Save your money.

One final word about ketones. People will tell you that producing ketones is dangerous for the body. This is just misinformation. They are confusing the ketogenic diet with ketoacidosis, which occurs in uncontrolled diabetics. This diet does NOT produce ketoacidosis.

Ketones may have two bad side effects. The first is the ketone headache. When you begin a ketogenic diet, or when you fast without food or water, the ketones can build up to a level that can affect the brain. The brain can use ketones as fuel, but it normally doesn't get many ketones. It's like a factory that makes apple juice. Squeezing the fruit, and filtering it, is geared to handling apples. Suppose there were no more apples, but a convoy of trucks came by carrying grapes. It shouldn't take long to convert that factory to efficiently handle the grapes to make grape juice, but it will take a short period of adjustment to tool up for the special processes that efficient squeezing of the grapes will need. It's the same with the brain. It can handle ketones, but it takes a day or two for the machinery to gear up to handle the load. During that time you may get the ketotic headache. It goes away all by itself. Drinking plenty of liquids helps, and if all else fails, an over-the-counter headache pill will work. Even when fully on the diet, if you don't drink enough water, you can get an occasional ketotic headache. Indeed, that is one of the self-tests for adequate fluid intake.

The other side effect as mentioned above is the acetone breath. Again, drinking enough fluid should dilute this effect to a minimal level. How much fluid intake is adequate? Probably no less than 6 - 8 glasses of water per day. This can be made up with water, pop, and tea, coffee and other drinks. However, be aware that caffeine is a diuretic and will cause the kidneys to get rid of fluids. Try to drink decaffeinated or caffeine-free beverages most of the time. However, if you must have your morning "Java," its OK.

The ketones have one or two very pleasant side effects. They give you a sense of well-being and they suppress your appetite. So the less carbohydrate you eat, the higher the level of your ketosis and the less you will want to eat.

One high carbohydrate meal will remove all of the ketones from your body very rapidly. It can take a day or two to get back to where you were. Since you won't have the ketones, you will probably eat more and stop your weight loss, at least temporarily. If you eat two or more consecutive high carbohydrate meals, you will start the weight piling back on and you must return to the first phase transition diet to get back on track. Even if this happens, don't lose faith in yourself. Sure you had a moment of weakness, but you did it once and you can get back on track.

Unlimited Energy

The other great benefit of the diet reported by all the research subjects was their increased energy levels. No more afternoon "crashes". No more crawling home after work and falling asleep in the chair after dinner. This diet gives something that no low calorie or low fat diet can provide. It provides an unlimited source of energy. You will have to experience it yourself in order to believe that dietary modifications alone can produce such a dramatic change in your alertness and mood.

Why do you have to go through the first phase transition diet? Theoretically, you don't, but it may take a longer time for your body to change to a fat burning machine during which time you may give into temptation and lose your motivation for the diet. The purpose of the transition diet is to deprive the body of almost all carbohydrates and force it to switch over to burning fat for fuel as quickly as possible. This requires totally different enzyme machinery than the carbohydrate factories. Once your body is convinced that the carbohydrates are not coming back, it will put all its efforts into creating enough capacity to satisfy all your energy needs from fats. That means not only the very efficient handling of dietary fats, but also the ability to mobilize that fat reserve its been carefully sculpting on your thighs, waist and hips for the past few years. It's as though your body has been saving for a rainy day and it has just started to pour. Once all this machinery is in place, you have turned your body into a fat burning furnace. Need some energy? Take it from my butt. Need more energy? Take it from my thigh. Your enzyme machinery can handle large quantities of dietary fat, and it now has the ability to mobilize your entire fat stores. You no longer have to put the feedbag on to get energy. You have it on demand, gushing forth from your fat cells like a newly-found oil well.

One of our research subjects told us that she looked forward to doing housework when she got home. She felt so good that she even dusted off the fifteen years of dust accumulation from her ironing board. Now we can't promise that you will enjoy ironing, but you should see this increase in daily stamina. All other forms of weight loss dieting tend to leave you with low energy reserves.

More lab results

At the end of the fourth week, our subjects returned for another fasting blood test battery. They did this every four weeks until the end of the study. Everyone was anxious to see his or her cholesterol results. After all, they had always been told to cut their fat intake and we were forcing a high fat diet on them. The results were remarkable. In general, there was over a 50% reduction in their fasting triglycerides. This showed that the conversion to a fat burning machine really worked. People who have problems with their serum triglyceride levels are classified as having type IV or type IIb lipoproteinemia. We have known for decades that this is a carbohydrate-induced condition. That message seems to have gotten lost with the high carbohydrate, low fat diet craze of the nineties. Our subjects, although they had normal triglycerides at the beginning of the study, nevertheless demonstrated that most of the triglycerides in the blood have nothing to do with dietary fat intake. They are the product of carbohydrate metabolism. What happened to our one subject with the 800 triglyceride? At four weeks into the diet, this subject had a fasting triglyceride of 170 mg/dL. That response is just what a doctor would like to see, and it is a response seen without drugs, with diet alone.

There was little change in the LDL cholesterol levels and HDL levels at four weeks. Thus, the high fat and high dietary cholesterol intake (at least by today's standards) did not cause the subjects any harm in their blood lipids. However, there was improvement in the subjects who had elevated liver enzymes. By the end of the 12 week study, every subject had normal liver enzyme results. All other tests did not change significantly and confirmed that nutritional markers did not worsen in any way on this diet.

As the diet progressed week after week, the story did not change with regard to the way the subjects felt about the diet. Finally, at the end of the 12 weeks, we had significant reduction in the total cholesterol and triglycerides with a small reduction in the LDL cholesterol which is associated with cardiac risk. The HDL (or "good" cholesterol) levels remained, on average, unchanged. So, the diet tended to reduce the cardiac risk associated with total and LDL cholesterol. But, at that point, the diet by itself did not raise protective HDL cholesterol levels nor did it lower HDL. (We have looked into this issue of modifying LDL cholesterol and raising HDL cholesterol and feel that increasing fiber, garlic, and vitamin E in the diet may help as well as promoting exercise. It can be done by diet choices. More about that later.)

What about weight loss?

Yes, our subjects did lose weight (otherwise there would be no purpose for this book). The range of weight loss for the 24 subjects who completed the 12 week study was from a low of four pounds to a high of 45 pounds. The average weight loss at 12 weeks was around 20 pounds, which was about a 10% reduction in body weight for this group. Not bad for a diet without much hardship.

Remember by comparison, a recent dietary miracle drug you've seen on TV promises weight losses of <10% after ONE YEAR of use. And it has side effects of bloating, diarrhea, and fecal incontinence.

The weight loss was not linear. No one lost two pounds per week, every week. Some weeks there was no weight loss and other weeks there was remarkable weight loss. Those little plateaus were discouraging to the subjects, but analysis of their food intake could usually provide a reason. One cheated at her son's birthday party. Another cheated at a beer and pizza party. Others found less obvious causes. One subject had severe arthritis and was put on non-steroidal anti-inflammatory drugs by her own physician. That was the end of the weight loss for that subject. Several of the post-menopausal women who were taking hormone replacement therapy had the slowest weight loss. They still lost weight and they still had all the positive feelings while on the diet. Their loss was just slower. Men lost the same average weight as women. There was no predictor that could forecast who would loose the most weight. Not even calorie intake affected the results. The subject who lost the most weight ate an average of 1200 calories per day, but the runner up ate 2600 calories per day. The point is that everyone is an individual and will respond to the diet in their own way and at their own rate. Importantly, all weight loss came from fat stores. Since we measured each subject's waist and hip dimensions at the beginning and end of the study, we were able to see an average of 5 inches lost in the waist, precisely where you would expect to find fat loss.

An exit poll conducted at the end of the study showed no negative comments. Everyone felt better. Everyone lost some weight. Everyone lost inches in the waist. And everyone now knew how he or she could solve their own weight problem successfully. What were the beneficial effects most cited apart from the weight loss?

- No more bloating after a meal.

- No need for antacids. Digestion improved.

- Abundant energy.

- Food no longer played a central role in life.

- Fewer vague aches and pains.

Our conclusion was that this diet was well-received and easy to comply with. The high monounsaturated fat levels did indeed protect all the subjects from rising cholesterol and the low carbohydrates alleviated many of the problems of hyperinsulinemia and insulin resistance. From additional observations and personal experience over the longer haul, we found that we could make additional changes such as lowering the LDL cholesterol with garlic and increasing fiber and raising the HDL cholesterol with vitamin E naturally or with supplements. Although these issues were not deliberately stressed in the original diet plan, they may offer additional benefits of dietary modification.

Thus we have **The Goldberg-O'Mara Diet.**

Chapter Four:
Science and the Diet

Some people are just fat, but others show a whole bunch of related problems. "Syndrome X" also known as "insulin resistance syndrome" or the "metabolic syndrome" is defined by these features:

- Resistance to insulin-mediated glucose uptake
- Glucose intolerance
- Hyperinsulinemia
- Increased very low density lipoprotein triglycerides (VLDL)
- Decreased high-density lipoprotein cholesterol (HDL)
- Hypertension
- Elevated systolic blood pressure during submaximal exercise
- Increased fat mass

The inherited defect is presumed to be insulin resistance in skeletal muscles and the other abnormalities are consequences. However, modern techniques of statistical analysis suggest there may not be one central abnormality, but a series of interlinked events leading to the syndrome. Whatever the cause, you will find that this diet relieves most of the symptoms of this syndrome.

You may start this diet if you are otherwise a healthy person. But if you have any associated diseases or have a strong family history of cardiac disease, diabetes, or hypertension, you should have medical screening first. For those people, we would strongly suggest you get the basic lab work done before you embark on this new lifestyle. Ask your physician or health clinic for a full lipid profile, glucose, and creatinine analysis. Although it is not commonly ordered, your doctor may also want to do a fasting insulin level.

Most labs and doctors will ask you for a fasting specimen for all of the above tests. However, lipid analysis can be more diagnostic if you get the blood drawn within two to three hours after you eat a low fat, high carbohydrate breakfast, such as cereal with skimmed milk, bagel or toast with jelly, fruit, juice, etc. And, please do not drink any alcohol at least 24 hours before the test. The LDL and HDL cholesterol levels are not affected much by the non-fasting state but the rate of clearance of triglycerides and the conversion of sugar into fats which remain in the circulation for long times will be picked up by this "postprandial" test. (Postprandial is medicalese for "after eating").

The fasting blood tests are also useful for monitoring results of the diet. What results do we look for? The National Cholesterol Education Program has recommended the following guidelines for lipid screening:

- Total cholesterol should be less than 200 mg/dL.

- HDL cholesterol should be greater than 29mg/dL in men and 38 in women. (Note: if the HDL-cholesterol is over 60mg/dl, it is felt to be a protective factor in cardiac disease, that is, a <u>negative</u> risk factor)

- Triglycerides should be less than 200 mg/dL

- LDL cholesterol should be less than 130 mg/dL (And if you have a history of angina or known coronary artery disease or a heart attack, the LDL should be less than 100 mg/dl)

If your LDL is high without an elevation in the triglycerides, this diet may or may not reduce your cholesterol levels even though it reduces your weight. Pushing garlic and fiber in the diet may help, but, if after a 2 – 3 month trial of the diet, a repeat analysis of the serum lipids does not show improvement, you should seek treatment from your physician to benefit from additional cholesterol-lowering drugs. Again, this diet will not make the LDL worse, but it may not be enough for you to lose weight alone in order to reduce this cardiac risk factor.

If your triglycerides are high and your HDL cholesterol is below 35 mg/dl, you will greatly benefit from this diet. You are the probably one of the Syndrome X people. Even if your HDL was normal, you may still have Fredrickson's Type IV lipoproteinemia. These syndromes are very carbohydrate-sensitive and this diet should normalize your serum lipids.

If your report mentions that your serum was milky and your triglyceride level was in the thousands, you should seek medical intervention. This condition can be due to a variety of causes including alcoholism, obesity, diabetes mellitus, uremia, nephrotic syndrome, pancreatitis, glycogen storage diseases, drugs such as steroids, and many more. The diet may help you, but it should be followed under strict medical supervision to prevent any undesirable side effects. The exact biochemical defect is still unknown, both for this condition and the Syndrome X, but it may be due to reduction in the enzymes which break down fats in the blood (lipoprotein lipases) or to defective mechanisms of removal of the lipoprotein particles, or to both. One theory suggests a possible influence of insulin on the production of a lipoprotein particle called apo C-III. This particle has an inhibitory effect on lipoprotein and hepatic lipases, the enzymes which breakdown the fat in the triglyceride containing lipoproteins. Since the **Goldberg-O'Mara Diet** has been shown to lower insulin and cause dramatic falls in serum triglyceride levels, this would certainly be supportive of this theory.

WHY "LOW CARBOHYDRATE"?
The Role of Insulin
Why do "very low calorie" and "low fat" diets fail in obese subjects almost one hundred percent of the time? Sure the subjects lose weight, but most of these dieters end up heavier than when they started the diet and they regain their weight within a year. What drives their bodies back up the scale? We're sure many of you have been in this boat. Alas, you were doomed to failure even before you started. No weight loss clinic or diet pill yet invented can cure your basic disease. Yes, we did say "disease". You have a chronic illness and until you face that fact, you're not going to get well (slim). You have tried treating the symptoms (your weight problem), but until you treat your underlying disease there will be no permanent results. You are driven to self-treat your disease by the only thing your body wants. We're talking about sugar. Otherwise healthy, fat people in general suffer from a condition called "hyperinsulinism". That means they produce more insulin to normalize blood sugar levels than thin people. The scientific literature is crammed full of research papers describing this event. There is nothing new about it. So why has it been ignored by mainstream medical practice? It is probably because the problem of weight was not epidemic in our society until recently. In that same time frame, we have become preoccupied with a bystander called cholesterol who just happened to be in the wrong place at the wrong time. Over the past 25 years, we have had a constant barrage of propaganda imploring, cajoling and threatening us to cut out fats and red meat from our diet and eat more carbohydrates, especially complex carbohydrates.

The message was simple and food processors and agribusiness benefitted. Carbohydrates in processed foods are relatively much cheaper than proteins. Couple this fact with the observations that carbohydrates tend to have an addictive quality about them. Not exactly like heroin or nicotine. But if you eat more carbohydrates, you will produce more insulin which will cause your blood sugar to fall, which will make you hungry and so you will eat more carbohydrates. Inadvertently, a vicious cycle was being established. We were told to eat less fats and meats. So, what did the market provide us with to eat? More carbohydrates.

This cycle of sugar-insulin-more sugar-more insulin starts off pretty innocently. Most people can handle it. They have the genetic makeup to adapt to this type of diet. You know the type. They sit opposite you in the cafeteria shoveling carbohydrate rich foods down their gullet. Their trays are overflowing with food. Yet they are skinny. Not slim, but really skinny. Boy, don't you hate those people? But there is also a substantial minority that can take it for only so long. Their tissues get tired of sugar highs with increased circulating insulin levels, so their cells go through a process call "down regulation". This results in the insulin having less of an effect on the cells. The pancreas, which produces the insulin, doesn't get the feedback to switch off the insulin production. So, increasingly more insulin is produced.

This forms a vicious cycle leading to two conditions. One is called insulin resistance and the other is hyperinsulinemia. If you have the appropriate genes and you get into this cycle, there is only one outcome. Type 2 diabetes. Over 80% of Type 2 diabetics are overweight and a substantial proportion of fat people will become diabetic.

Some of us become hyperinsulinemic early in life. Babies born to mothers who were uncontrolled diabetics are hyperinsulinemic, and apart from being very large babies due to the effect of this hyperinsulinism, they also become heavy later in life. Others become hyperinsulinemic at the onset of puberty, become fat adolescents, thin out for early adulthood then go into their middle age spread.

What is happening? What does control of blood sugar have to do with my being fat?

To answer this question we must get a little technical. First, think of hormones as e-mail and receptors as e-mail addresses. Insulin is a hormone (E-mail) produced by the pancreas. Its main claim to fame is in diabetes due to its function in controlling blood sugars. But that isn't the only effect of insulin. Many tissues have insulin receptors (E-mail addresses which will accept the E-mail) and the function of insulin varies with the tissue. In muscle cells, the insulin is mainly concerned with causing the cells to take glucose out of the bloodstream and to put it into storage as a molecule called glycogen. Glycogen is animal starch. It is a huge molecule made by linking many glucose molecules together. As the blood sugar falls, there is too much E-mail, and the cells respond by closing their mail boxes. This creates a feedback loop to the pancreas to stop producing the hormone.

The main storage organ for sugar is the liver. The insulin effect on these liver cells may not be downregulated to the same degree in hyperinsulinemia as it is in muscle cells. It means that if you are hyperinsulinemic and eat a big pasta meal with plenty of garlic bread, followed by pie or ice cream dessert you are going to suffer. The better it tasted going down, the more you will get that bloating about one hour to two hours later. Your pancreas is producing insulin as fast as its little enzyme factory can work and although you muscle cells may be resistant, your liver is just stuffing those sugar molecules into glycogen until the cells begin to swell. The excess sugar is then converted into fat and stored in the liver. Your liver gets so big you think you are going to burst. The process is relentless.

While the liver is producing its glycogen, it is also *converting all excess sugar* into fatty acids which are exported into the blood stream and carried to the fat cells for storage. And the fat cells also come under the influence of those high insulin levels which urges them to remove the fats and more glucose from the blood and store everything as body fat.

Once things calm down, the liver starts exporting the fat which is then carried by protein packets called lipoproteins. The one, which carries the fat away from the liver, is called VLDL. This lipoprotein travels in the blood stream until it reaches target tissues that produce enzymes, called lipases, to break down these fats and release fatty acids. This happens in the arterial walls and in fat tissue. The remnant VLDL particles can then go through a series of interactions with other lipoproteins in the plasma and after taking on a load of cholesterol become particles called LDL. It is these cholesterol rich LDL particles, especially those damaged by what are called "free radicals", which can be deposited in the arterial walls leading to atherosclerosis. In diabetics, and probably in obesity, the VLDL remnant particle itself may be deposited in the artery wall. This is probably why most type 2 diabetics die from coronary artery disease and not from the other deleterious effects of diabetes. As we have already discussed, obesity and diabetes are kissing cousins.

Slowly, as your blood sugar falls, the pancreas slows down and produces less insulin, and starts to release another hormone called "glucagon" but the process tends to overshoot the mark in fat people due to the hyperinsulinemia. Your blood sugars fall too far or too fast probably because the balancing hormone, glucagon, can't work properly in the presence of all this insulin. This can cause symptoms of hypoglycemia, but in most cases it will simply cause the person to go look for food. In a normal individual, the insulin levels would fall away to very low levels and as your blood sugar dropped, your liver, under the influence of glucagon, would start releasing sugar from it's stored glycogen, and the fat cells would release their fats after all the glycogen was used up. This would stabilize the blood sugar and there would be little feeling of hunger for many hours. The obese hyperinsulinemic individual has too much circulating insulin, which inhibits this natural process, and we get hungry. So we go looking for food. And we are not looking for carrots or celery sticks. These types of foods are not going to solve our immediate problem of falling sugars. We are driven to eat foods that will relieve our symptoms. That means a carbohydrate snack. A couple of cookies, a bag of pretzels, a slice of cake or pie. That is what makes us feel better.

Yes, the problem is driven by insulin, and unless and until we address that problem, the weight is going to stay with us. There is nothing else it can do. That's nature and you can't fight Mother Nature. You can now see why the low fat, high carbohydrate diets don't work for you. Carbohydrates defeat everything you are trying to accomplish. You must be ready and willing to face your problem and GIVE UP ALL HIGH CARBOHYDRATE FOODS. You need to keep your net carbohydrates below the threshold that will stimulate increasingly higher insulin release.

It's not as bad as it sounds. We didn't say you couldn't have any carbohydrates. You simply need to follow a "low carbohydrate" lifestyle. What we mean by low carbohydrate lifestyle is not eating any food that contains more than three or four grams of NET CARBOHYDRATE per serving. All vegetables contain some carbohydrate. In most cases, it is indigestible fiber, so it doesn't count. What counts are sugars and starches. They are your "poisons".

Stay away from any processed cereal grains and flours and anything made from milled flours. That means no conventional breads, cereals, cookies, or pastas. Stay away from starchy vegetables. That means no potatoes, beans, peas, lentils and corn. Stay away from sugars. That means no sugar itself or in any form such as candies, sweets, sodas, puddings, milk and nearly all fruit. These are the foods that prevent your cells from giving up their fat. Until you reach your desired weight, that is a commandment. There must be no cheating.

Right now you may be saying "I can't do this". Wrong, Wrong, Wrong. We've done it. Dozens upon dozens of people have now done it. You can do it and you must do it. It is your salvation. When you start the diet, the feelings of deprivation will last no more than three to four days. From then on you will not crave any of the high carbohydrate foods. That doesn't mean you won't miss them. You won't crave them, therefore you will have the willpower to resist eating them.

WHY "HIGH MONOUNSATURATED FATS"?

By now, everyone has heard of the association between fats containing saturated fatty acids and heart disease, cancer, and possibly diabetes. All of the studies were based on diets that were high in saturated fat but also, relatively high in carbohydrate content. To date, we have not found any study showing the effects of reasonable amounts of saturated fats on people who eat a diet low in carbohydrate content. But we are taking a conservative approach with this and will continue to recommend, for the present at least, put a *limit on saturated fat.*

As you may know, your plasma <u>cholesterol</u> level is much more dependent on your fat consumption than on your cholesterol intake when you consume a diet high in carbohydrate. Most people (about 70%) will reduce their plasma cholesterol levels dramatically if they eat a very low carbohydrate diet. There are numerous books and papers published on the effects of the hunter-gatherer type diet. Tribal peoples who eat only meat, fish, and the few seasonal vegetables, nuts and fruits, in their habitat tend to have low incidences of heart disease and diabetes. The point of the tribal diet is that while it is high fat, the diets are simultaneously low in carbohydrates.

One author of a popular low carbohydrate diet book does warn that about 30% of people will be fat-sensitive and their cholesterol will go up if they eat his diet. However, we have found in the literature and shown in our studies that the high consumption of monounsaturated fats can counteract this effect. There are numerous publications to justify this claim.

There is also evidence of a relationship between fatty acids and serum insulin. These researchers measured plasma phospholipid fatty acid levels, an indicator of fatty acid composition in the diet, and demonstrated levels that were associated with fasting serum insulin concentrations (a marker of insulin resistance). They examined 4,304 middle-aged adults free of diabetes. Fasting insulin was strongly and positively associated with the saturated fatty acid percentage in plasma phospholipids, moderately and inversely associated with the monounsaturated percentage, and not appreciably associated with the polyunsaturated fat percentage. These data are consistent with studies showing that fatty acid composition of cell membranes modulates insulin action, and support the hypothesis that increased habitual saturated fat intake or a related dietary pattern is a risk factor for hyperinsulinemia. It should follow that monounsaturated fats would relieve this problem.

Monounsaturated fats also seem to provide a degree of protection against some cancers. One of the conclusions of a case-controlled study showed unsaturated fatty acids protect against breast cancer, possibly because intake of these nutrients is also closely correlated with a high intake of vegetables. The findings also suggested a possible increased risk of breast cancer in southern European populations whose diet largely based on starch (carbohydrates).

WHY "DIETARY FIBER"?

Fiber is plant material that is indigestible to humans. There are two main categories, soluble and insoluble. They are very complex carbohydrates digested by the bacteria which live in the intestines of insects like termites and herbivorous animals such as sheep and cows. We humans do not have these bacteria living in our digestive system, therefore, most dietary fiber will pass through our intestines unchanged. Some bacteria may break down some soluble fiber with gas production (the bean effect) but there is no evidence that we benefit from their action.

That does not mean that the fiber is useless. It can react with other things in our intestines with many beneficial effects. The first good effect is that fiber will hold water. This is the basis of the laxative function of many of the over-the-counter dietary aids to prevent or treat constipation. If you have enough fiber in your diet, your stools should remain bulky and soft. The second documented beneficial effect of high levels of dietary fiber is that it binds the cholesterol compounds secreted into the bile, keeping them from being reabsorbed into the blood. This has the effect of lowering blood cholesterol levels.

Fiber has also been implicated as having a protective effect against many cancers. A study on rats looked at this effect. Experimental and epidemiological evidence suggests that increased dietary fiber is associated with decreased breast cancer risk but little was known about the role played by different types of fiber, and particularly mixtures of soluble and insoluble fibers similar to those consumed by human populations, in reducing breast cancer risk. High intake of fiber may suppress bacterial breakdown of biliary estrogen conjugates to free (absorbable) estrogens in the colon and thus may decrease the availability of circulating estrogens necessary for the development and growth of breast cancers. The study evaluated the effect of wheat bran (an insoluble fiber) and psyllium (a soluble fiber) alone and in combination on overall estrogen status and on the induction of mammary tumors in rats treated with a cancer-causing agent. The results demonstrated that as the level of psyllium relative to that of wheat bran increased, the total tumor number and multiplicity of mammary tumors in rats decreased. The authors concluded that the addition of a 4%:4% mixture of an insoluble (wheat bran) fiber and a soluble (psyllium) fiber to a high-fat diet provided the maximum tumor-inhibiting effects in this breast tumor model. Although increasing levels of dietary psyllium were associated with decreased bacterial enzyme activity, these changes were not reflected in decreased circulating levels of tumor-promoting estrogens. Therefore, the mechanism(s) by which mixtures of soluble and insoluble dietary fibers protect against mammary tumorigenesis still remains to be clarified.

WHY "KEFIR, YOGURT AND OTHER FERMENTED MILK PRODUCTS"?

Lactobacillus and similar organisms are the bacteria that convert milk to products like buttermilk, cheese, yogurt and kefir. They are also plentiful in a healthy human bowel and are the normal organisms in the female's vagina. However, our modern diets and consumption of drugs, especially antibiotics, can disrupt the normal bacterial colonization. This can lead to many gastrointestinal complaints and vaginal infections. A steady source of live lactobacillus organisms in the diet will help maintain a healthy bowel and help prevent overgrowth of the bowel and the vagina by such organisms as Candida albicans, a notorious yeast whose presence can give many vague symptoms. Needless to say, this is not the book to discuss this subject, but we do recommend daily intake of at least 1/2-1 cup of live culture kefir, yogurt or buttermilk daily as a method to constantly replenish your lactobacillus.

As mentioned earlier, the milk fermenting organisms have recently been found to stimulate the immune system and keeping the immune system in tune is probably key to the body's natural defenses against infectious diseases and cancer. This research has shown that among its many good qualities, these bacteria also stimulate the body to produce important immune response chemicals called "cytokines". These "might promote a continuous state of alertness against attack by viruses and other pathogenic organisms," according to one study.

If you think you can't take milk products because you are lactase deficient, don't worry! People who can't tolerate milk because it causes bloating and diarrhea have these symptoms because their bodies cannot break down the lactose in milk. DON'T WORRY ABOUT THIS with kefir and yogurt. The lactobacillus in the kefir or yogurt will produce enough enzymes to destroy most of the remaining lactose and convert it into lactic acid. With the breakdown of lactose by these good bacteria, you can enjoy these products daily (and SHOULD as part of a healthy lifestyle). It is important that you choose a reliable maker of your kefir or yogurt and that your product contains live cultures.

Lactic acid (produced by the bacteria's breakdown of lactose) happens to be a very powerful natural antimicrobial and may protect you somewhat from Salmonella and Shigella food poisoning. Indeed, consumption of a daily breakfast containing kefir or yogurt while traveling may even protect you from many of the causes of traveler's diarrhea.

More science

The scientific literature is profuse with research papers, each contributing a small piece of the puzzle, but when combined they present a deafening condemnation of the some of the nutritional advice currently advocated by governmental and academic societies. Why have those august bodies not modified their positions? It is not because these papers were published in obscure journals. Indeed, most of them have been published in the most prestigious journals of the medical profession. It is not because the research results are in doubt. Rather, it is probably an inability to admit that the advice so freely administered may be contributing to the epidemics of obesity and Type 2 diabetes which we see today. Yes, the "heart friendly diets" may be fine for a majority of the population, perhaps even a big majority, but what about the misery caused to the 25 to 30 percent of the population it will harm?

What's the proof?

Well, let's work backwards for a couple of years just skimming the reports.

In November of 1997, *The New England Journal of Medicine* published a paper which demonstrated that moderate restriction of dietary fat intake achieved meaningful and sustained LDL cholesterol reductions in hypercholesterolemic subjects (HC) and apolipoprotein B reductions in both hypercholesterolemic and subjects with combined hypercholesterolemia (CHL) and hypertriglyceridemia. Their conclusions were that "more extreme restriction of fat intake offers little further advantage in HC or CHL subjects and potentially undesirable effects in HC subjects". These authors demonstrated that lowering the fat content below the 30% of calories actually causes harm. Did they question whether 30% fat calories and 50 to 60% carbohydrate calories was a diet suitable for hypertriglyceridemic subjects even although they all remained or became hypertriglyceridemic while on the diet? No.

A paper in the *American Journal of Clinical Nutrition* demonstrated an increase from 8 percent to 13 percent in the number of women with an undesirable (that means <u>low</u>) HDL cholesterol after the American Heart Association diet intervention. These authors write "a decline in the HDL-cholesterol concentration in response to a high carbohydrate, low-fat diet is potentially harmful for older women who are at a heightened risk for coronary artery disease". They also state "a low-fat diet without substantial weight loss is not beneficial for improving lipoprotein lipid risk factors in obese, postmenopausal women with normal lipid profiles". These authors had the insight to comment that "Weight loss <u>without</u> a low-fat diet may increase HDL cholesterol above pretreatment values while also lowering total cholesterol". Did anyone hear of this study on the nightly news broadcast? Why not?

A second study involving only ten individual subjects published in the same journal confirmed these findings and showed that these "untoward metabolic effects of low-fat, high carbohydrate diets are directly related to degree of insulin resistance". Therefore, women who are overweight to begin with are most likely to increase their risk factors for heart disease by eating a high carbohydrate diet.

This phenomenon is not limited to postmenopausal women. A paper published in the journal, *Pediatrics,* also concluded "not only that obese adolescents have lipid abnormalities (elevated serum LDL-C and triglycerides, and reduced HDL-C levels) but also that these abnormalities correlate with the degree of insulin resistance". Again we see the link between obesity, insulin resistance and serum lipid abnormalities. Are you beginning to get the picture?

Let's go back to an even earlier age. Caprio, and co-researchers clearly demonstrate that insulin resistance and hyperinsulinemia co-exist in adolescent children with moderate to severe obesity. There are papers that go all the way back to the effects of hyperinsulinism of the fetus caused by gestational diabetes. The story is always the same. Golay and associates studied forty-three adult obese subjects who were assigned to either a high carbohydrate (45%) or a low carbohydrate (15%) low calorie diet. The weight loss was about the same for both groups after six weeks. However, the low carbohydrate diet group had significantly lower insulin, cholesterol and triglyceride levels at the end of the test period. These authors concluded that "consumption of the kind of low fat, high carbohydrate diet for weight maintenance advocated by the National Cholesterol Education Program seems to minimize the fall in plasma insulin and triacylglycerol concentrations". Again, more proof that the <u>high</u> fat, <u>low</u> carbohydrate diets may be better for weight loss programs. Of course this study emphasized calorie restriction. **The Goldberg-O'Mara Diet** finds that if we keep the carbohydrates low, we can increase the fat intake while maintaining the weight loss. Of course, the right kinds of fats are key.

Perhaps one of the most telling, yet underreported papers was published in the prestigious *Journal of Pediatrics*. These authors studied fruit juice intake in one hundred and sixteen 2-year-olds and one hundred and seven 5-year-old children. They demonstrated that 2 year olds who drank more than 12 fluid ounces of fruit juice per day were three times as likely as their peers (47% versus 14%) to be short. Also, the juice drinkers had thirty two percent of children with a BMI greater than the ninetieth percentile for BMI versus only nine percent for children who drank less than twelve fluid ounces of juice per day.

Does this mean that drinking excess fruit juices caused these children to be short and fat? This was not proved by this study. It does bring up the interesting observation that our body's natural satiety (feeling of satisfaction) from real fruit is bypassed when you drink fruit juice. You probably would not eat more than one orange or apple at a time if you were eating the whole fruit, right? But you think nothing of consuming the juice from three, four or maybe even five oranges or apples when you drink a tall glass of juice. You drink all of the carbohydrates and get almost none of the fiber!

Those of you who are old enough may remember that before the nineteen-sixties, apples and oranges were tart. Slowly, but surely, agribusiness has bred out the tartness and left or increased the sweetness of all fruit. After all, you can sell many more sweet oranges than tart oranges. They have bypassed our natural ability to say "No more! I am satisfied." You older guys can also remember that fruit used to be only seasonally available. Oranges were available for only a few months. Strawberries were the treat of early summer. And bananas were only imported during short growing seasons. Now, with the improvement of transportation systems, refrigeration and multinational agribusiness, we can get almost any fruit or vegetable all year round. When you walk into your super-market, it is perpetual summer. Never in the history of mankind has this happened and the result is seen in your hips and waist. We can now feed our hyperinsulinism with so-called, nutritious fruits and their juices all year round.

One of the newest papers at the time of publishing the current edition of this book is a study from the journal *Pediatrics* by Willi and others who demonstrated rapid weight loss in adolescents with little loss in lean body weight. Again, they clearly demonstrate the safety of very low carbohydrate diets, even in children twelve to fifteen years old.

So why would anyone feed a high carbohydrate diet to anyone with hyperinsulinism? Is the defect reversible by continually stimu-lating the pancreas to produce more insulin? Why do the scientists and clinicians continually confuse the well-documented bad effects of a high fat and high carbohydrate diet with the clearly demon-strated benefits of a very low carbohydrate diet?

Everyone should agree that the first priority to treat obesity is normalizing the weight. Low carbohydrate diets do this effectively and quickly and if you follow the **Goldberg-O'Mara Diet**, without increasing any of the lipid risk factors. What to do long term may be debated for years to come. We have no prospective scientific data on the long-term effects of a very low carbohydrate diet except for anecdotal reports. The assumption is that a return to high carbohy-drate intake will produce the same effect as it did originally in those individuals who gained weight on high carbs before. So, *we suggest that eating low carbohydrates with the appropriate modifications of high monounsaturated fats, high fiber, natural sources of vitamins, minerals, antioxidants, and phytochemicals through several servings of assorted vegetables each day, and fermented milk products will have to be a permanent dietary change.* But, can you even think that your former eating habits gave you as much nutrition?

Still, we will have to monitor benefits in the years to come to see if nutrition can promote health over a lifetime. This will be hard. After all, would you really want to go back to your old way of eating and risk the return to weight gain and its associated diseases? It would be hard to get volunteers to agree to do a crossover study.

A word about exercise.

We spoke briefly about the evidence that exercising as little as brisk walking daily may have a positive effect on raising HDL (good) cholesterol. We strongly support exercise by brisk walking, starting with ten minutes a day and working up to 20-30 minutes. A general program of mobility exercising is also advisable. However, you should be doing this exercise for its benefits on the general conditioning of the body and for possible effects on raising HDL cholesterol. You should NOT exercise for the purpose of weight loss. The diet is for weight loss.

During our study, we specifically forbade the subjects from starting an exercise program concurrent with the diet study. Why? We wanted to look strictly at the effects of the diet upon weight loss and biochemical markers in the blood. Weight loss from exercise, as we said in Chapter 2, is minimal. Let the diet work for weight loss. If you are significantly overweight, attempting to increase exercise beyond walking may be harmful to you. Yes, we said harmful. We feel that any exercise program beyond simple brisk walking should be medically supervised. We support exercise when and how it is recommended by your doctor. You'll get there, but at the right pace, safely.

Chapter Five:
Healthy Eating for a Healthy Life

It may seem trite to say, "you are what you eat", but in many ways it's true. The previous chapter on **Science and the Diet** has shown you that what you eat may unmask or promote certain disease states. The evidence is convincing to show that obesity and its attendant relationships to cardiac disease, type 2 diabetes and hypertension may all be connected through the composition of our diets and their effects upon our underlying genetics. Also, we can worsen our diseases with certain diets and perhaps help them with others, such as the **Goldberg-O'Mara Diet.**

There is also no question as to the effects upon the sense of energy seen in those who have been following this diet. Let us relate a common anecdote we have heard over and over from our study participants and others who have subsequently used the diet. It had become a habit for many people to seek a nap, somewhere around 4 or 5 o'clock in the afternoon. People explained this phenomenon away by their age or workload or stress levels. Yet, almost without exception, the need for an afternoon nap completely disappeared within a week of starting the diet. This predated any serious weight loss. The only reason for having more energy and no longer seeking an afternoon nap could be attributed to the composition of the diet. We now laugh about it, yet we were previously resigned to "needing" extra rest. Changing our diet away from excessive carbo-hydrates had an impact upon our "need" for extra daytime sleep. And with it went the concept that we were just getting older and needed naps. Many people claimed that the diet gave them 10 years back and this was before the loss of weight and inches around the middle.

Of course, the psychological benefits of weight loss are unbeat-able for self-esteem. Our study subjects were mainly employees at the hospital in which we both worked so we were able to follow-up with their success as their weight loss continued after the study period. The original group recruited even more of their friends and families and, of course, we gave the diet freely to anyone who asked. So, we received a great deal of success stories and actually saw the process happening in many others. It was so nice to see the technician who was 200 pounds get down to 135 pounds over 9 months. It was good to hear about the diabetic sister of one of our study participants who went on the diet with her doctor's supervision. She went from using 95 units of insulin daily to using an oral agent only. How about one of our doctors who has thrown out 5 progressively smaller belts in the last six months as he has shed 56 pounds? He proudly wears shirts tucked in when he used to wear only scrub tops to work.

We see turtlenecks being worn under lab coats now, something impossible to do when there was a previous fat layer in-between. We and our fellow dieters have thrown or given away dowdy clothes in favor of more trendy cuts and shorter hemlines. No one fears summer. We have seen many examples of the transforming effect of weight loss and, indeed, it sometimes feels like we have been given back 10 years of our lives.

In August of 1998, our research was presented at a national meeting in Chicago. The local news station, Channel 2, picked up the story as part of their own series on diets. We were interviewed by Dr. Michael Breen, a highly respected physician-journalist, who caught onto the concepts of the diet immediately. A very short segment of video was run on the news over the next couple of days. The response to the story was overwhelming. Over 17,000 people requested the diet after seeing the brief story on television. Copies of our diet were distributed and we set up a website in order to reach more people. As part of our website, we set up a "virtual" support group. Between the website and mailings, we have received hundreds of testimonials from people who have used the diet.

Many of the stories followed the same theme. People had "dieted" for years, gradually becoming resigned to being overweight for life. Imagine their surprise when, for the first time, a diet actually produced weight loss without any penalties. People wrote to us about losing weight and buying new clothes for the first time in years, and in much lower dress sizes than they had ever expected! They told us of lowered weights and lowered cholesterols. They told us about having energy to do things after work. They told us about their new body images and feelings they now have about themselves.

One of our casual dieters, an emergency physician at a busy Chicago-area hospital, started the diet in January, 1998 and lost 80 pounds by the end of the year. During this time he also quit smoking (something he had done once before in the past), and was thrilled to find that he still lost weight, instead of gaining it. His enthusiasm was catchy. Several others in the Emergency department started the diet as a result of seeing his success with it. At the end of 1998, that Emergency department had lost some serious weight. When we were asked to appear in February, 1999 on WGN, Channel 9 in Chicago, they asked for someone who had been on the diet to share their story. Dr. Lewis was up for the challenge. The news team was skeptical of a high monounsaturated fat, low carbohydrate diet. Wasn't it going to be hard to follow and use alien foods? Image their surprise when he made lunch for them, homemade Cesear's salad and Chicken Cacciatore! The visit that was supposed to be just a few minutes lasted two and a half hours. His stories and luncheon showed the team how serious weight loss, by a method that promotes good eating habits, can impact one's life.

We believe that healthy eating can, and does, promote a healthy life. Health is composed of many factors: physical condition, sense of well- being, psychological state and all of these are improved when one is closer to their optimal weight. We now know that there is a significant role for the composition of the diet in influencing this outcome, too.

What is especially profound to us is the realization that we, and others, had made so many unintended errors in our previous treatments of weight loss. Errors like telling people to cut calories severely, to eat lots of cereals and "grains", or to rid their households of fats for a "sure" solution to their weight problem. Or telling forty- and fifty- year olds that they should expect weight gain because their metabolism was slowing down. Or telling younger people that they could just "exercise it all away". Some of these errors came from failing to question the recommendations of persons or organizations who were deemed to be "the experts".

The goal of modern medicine is to produce treatments that are "evidence-based". That means that there are appropriate studies showing reproducible outcomes that then justify a particular therapy. It seems in retrospect that we didn't demand a high level of evidence before accepting the old recommendations of our "experts". We now know that we must continuously question every aspect of our dietary research to assure that we are using the best possible, safest diet for whomever we treat. As clinicians, we must be diligent in seeking any and all scientific research that enables us to modify our diets in the future so that we can improve outcomes even more. While this diet has worked successfully for many otherwise healthy, overweight and more severely obese subjects, future research may point to new modifications for certain subgroups of patients with various medical conditions. This is why we must continuously emphasize that you **use this diet with your personal physician's oversight**, especially if you are under medical treatment for another condition.

Remember, too, that your doctor needs to be screening you for signs of other diseases in order to prevent problems in the future as we all age. So, while you're working hard on your weight, let your doctor help you by screening for other medical conditions, too.

Chapter Six: How to Shop

The two most difficult things at the beginning of the transition to eating on the **Goldberg-O'Mara Diet** are changing your mindset and re-tooling your pantry. No doubt your household is filled with everything "low fat" or "fat-free". Ours certainly were. When you stop to read the labels, it will become painfully obvious that many of the things in your kitchen cabinets and pantries are often incompatible with life on your new diet. So, let's start by looking at labels and then we can clean your cupboards out.

The "Nutrition Facts" Label

On the backs of every manufactured food sold will be a "Nutrition Facts" label. This label starts by giving the serving size. For example, a "serving" may be defined as "7 crackers" or "one ounce" or "2 slices". The "number of servings per container" will then be given. This is followed by "calories" and "calories from fat" which on this diet you can finally ignore. Next will be a table showing the "Amount per serving" of Total Fat (subdivisions of saturated fat and, sometimes monounsaturated and polyunsaturated fats are given), Cholesterol, Sodium, Total Carbohydrate (and the subdivisions, fiber and sugars), and Protein.

Let's look a little closer at the "Total Carbohydrate" and its subdivisions. This is the part of the label that is absolutely critical to read first. It will immediately tell you if you can even consider this food or not.

As you well know by now, you are limited to a total daily NET carbohydrate intake of 50 grams with only 12-15 grams of NET carbohydrate at any one meal. And EVERYTHING that might enter your mouth must be looked at for its carbohydrate content, whether it's solid or liquid, whether it's the meal or the dessert, whether it's the main course or a condiment, whether it's eaten standing up or sitting down. You get the picture.

"Total carbohydrates" per serving gives you all grams of sugars, starches, and fiber in that particular serving size of that particular food. However, in the subdivisions below the total, often only the fiber and sugar content are shown. If these two are added together, then subtracted from the total, the remainder will be starches.

Now we told you earlier that fiber is "free", that is, you don't have to count fiber in your total carbohydrate count. So, SUBTRACT THE GRAMS OF FIBER FROM THE <u>TOTAL</u> CARBOHYDRATE shown in order to get the <u>NET</u> CARBOHYDRATES which is the number in which we are interested.

Net Carbohydrates = Total Carbohydrates - Fiber

"Net Carbohydrates" is the amount that you are concerned about, the amount that must be counted into your carbohydrate allowance for that meal.

The "net carbohydrate" will be the amount of starches and sugars in that serving size of that particular food. Now you can decide if it's possible for you to eat that food or to use that product in your food preparation. How many grams are left? Are you willing to use your carbohydrate allowance for that meal on that food? Or, when all the math is done, is the result so high that you just can't eat any? You may be surprised to find that a lot of the processed foods in your old pantry meet that "JUST CAN'T EAT ANY" category.

Take a minute now and look at some of the food products in your pantry. Cereals made from milled flours often have carbohydrate counts that exceed the limit, so these will probably be out. But if you have a cereal with very high fiber, it may be okay. Do the math to find out. Cookie carbohydrate counts are obviously in excess. Check out the package labels for rice and couscous. The answer is the same, too high. Pretzels, rice cakes, snack crackers, potato chips and sticks, low fat snacks? Again, too many net carbs. Time to clean house. Don't feel badly. These things were driving your weight gain. They NEED to go.

So, processed foods will have to be carefully scrutinized before you buy anything. What's left to eat? Natural foods are going to have a better chance to work. Let's look at **Appendix One** at the end of the book to get a feel for the **Net Carbohydrate** count of many unprocessed foods. "Net carbohydrate" means that the fiber count has already been subtracted from the total.

In this appendix, and in subsequent carbohydrate counters that you may purchase or if you log onto the USDA website, be sure to PAY ATTENTION TO THE SERVING SIZE. In some cases, the serving size may represent more or less than what you would usually eat. You must multiply or divide accordingly to adjust for what size you would ACTUALLY eat. In our Appendix One, we have selected many foods that are low in net carbohydrates, even with very generous serving sizes. This list is a good place to start to pick out foods for your shopping list. You'll notice that potatoes, sweet potatoes, rice, pasta, peas, corn, pretzels, bagels, and bread are NOT listed. Let's think of substitutes for these foods from the approved foods.

Shopping Day

Start out with a shopping list. The following food lists are a good place to start and then modify and expand according to your tastes. This will not feel like previous diets. You will notice that the foods you will be eating are not "hardships". They are really good foods that you may have been avoiding. Let's take a look.

Condiments:
Mustard, horseradish, real mayonnaise, soy sauce, iodized salt, pepper, variety of cooking spices, spray and liquid canola oil, olive oil, salsa without sugar, guacamole, sugar-free, no calorie gelatin, sugar-free (diabetic) syrups

Vegetables:
Mixed greens, lettuce, radishes, onions, celery, cucumbers, collards, okra, green beans, wax beans, spinach, zucchini, spaghetti squash, summer squash, acorn squash, cauliflower, broccoli, Brussel sprouts, mushrooms, mixed Chinese vegetables. You can buy these fresh or frozen or canned provided there have been no added sugars. Buy plenty of variety and amount since you are expected to have 5 servings of vegetables a day. A serving size is roughly 1 cup of the raw vegetable.

Meats/Fish:
Fresh, unbreaded, lean poultry, beef, veal, pork. Fresh fish and shell-fish. Canned tuna , salmon and sardines in oil or water. Low saturated fat sausages and prepared luncheon meats. Remember to check that there are no added fillers in the sausages or meats. For vegetarians, check out soy and veggie-burgers.

Fruits:

Buy a VERY limited amount of fresh, unsweetened berries, kiwi, rhubarb or melons. or low sugar, tart apples or pears. Avoid frozen berries unless you are sure there is no sugar or syrup added. Remember your serving size is only 1/2 cup of ONE of these per day. Don't overbuy.

Dairy/Eggs/ Cheese:

Cultured, fermented milk products should be <u>first</u> on your list since we encourage 8 ounces of kefir or yogurt daily. Your Kefir and yogurt should have live cultures and be free of added starch or sugar.

Cheese blocks or cubes, string cheese, ricotta cheese, cream cheese, eggs, buttermilk, heavy cream. If you read labels closely, you may be able to find artificially sweetened yogurt without fruit that will be okay.

Cereal/Crackers:

Look very closely and don't get tricked by the labels. You CAN find the extremely high fiber bran cereal and high fiber, low "net carbo-hydrate" crispbread. Buy wheat bran, oat bran, and flaxseed. You may have to look especially hard at first to find these but it will be worth your effort for cooking your own pancakes and waffles and cereals.

Nuts and Seeds:

Pecans, almonds, macadamias, hazelnuts, walnuts, peanuts, edible seeds such as pumpkin seeds and sunflower seed kernels. Find the ones you like and buy these in bulk by the pound at wholesale stores for the freshest product and best prices.

Drinks:

Kefir, diet soda, diet powdered drinks, tea, coffee, light beer or dry wine, diet-only mixers.

What about those packaged foods that we've all become so dependent upon for convenience? Well sadly, many of those foods are excessively high in carbohydrate counts. When we need convenience, we have to start thinking differently. For example, think "rotissiere chicken and salad" instead of "frozen pizza". Both are available at most larger grocery stores. You just have to look at the deli sections now instead of the frozen food sections. Snacks become nuts and cheese instead of pretzels and rice cakes. No cookies or candy, instead buy sugar-free, flavored gelatin for use alone or with sugar-free whipped topping. No breakfast tarts or pre-made waffles. Instead, substitute high fiber crispbread with cream cheese and wheat bran waffles that you can make in advance and freeze, then pop in the toaster or microwave.

It may seem hard at first, but that is part of the education and re-tooling process. We have to make new, healthy eating habits replace the old habits that gave rise to an unhealthy (and fat) lifestyle. Once you have the proper ingredients and assortment of the right foods in the house, it's a lot easier. And we'll show you more in the next chapter on menu planning.

Chapter Seven:
Menu Suggestions

The most difficult part of any new diet is menu planning. Why? Because, it takes some thought. You can't rely on your old habits now. Menu planning moves the right foods into your daily life. It is your ACTION PLAN.

Menu planning is the key to success. If you do not have some organization, you will never have the proper ingredients on hand to prepare food that you will enjoy and that will enable you to comply with your diet. It's easy to revert back to old habits so be cautious of this temptation as you are re-tooling your pantry and re-thinking your menus. Sit down and plan what you will eat for the next week. Then make sure you have all of the necessary ingredients available.

Another good tip is to cook more than you need at the time, assuring yourself of a little "leftover". The leftovers can usually be frozen in single serve containers and make easy lunches that you can take to work or school. Heat them up in the office or cafeteria microwave oven and save money while sticking to your diet.

Another good idea is to cook extra meals on the weekends. You can also cook some foods, like wheat bran pancakes, in advance and freeze these in single serving packages. They microwave quickly and give you a good hot breakfast with sugar-free syrup and crushed pecans. You have created your own convenience food by cooking in bulk and freezing.

Rediscover some great kitchen cooking aids: the crockpot, the pressure cooker, and the electric skillet. Undoubtedly you have them hidden somewhere in the pantry. These can be lifesavers for the hectic household and will help you avoid convenience foods. Here are a few ideas to get you started.

For the crockpot:
- Start a pot roast with leeks, carrots, and celery in the morning and come home to a house filled with savory fragrances. Use a gravy enhancer, concentrated beef seasoning, and your favorite spices. Remember, in a crockpot, keep liquids to a minimum.

- Start chili with 2 pounds of pre-browned ground beef, chopped onions, celery and green pepper, 1 can of crushed tomatoes and chili seasonings to taste. Let it cook all day in the crockpot and dress it up with shredded cheese, sour cream and guacamole when you serve it.

- Put Italian sausages in the crockpot, cover with a few table-spoons of low carb seasoned tomato sauce or crushed tomatoes. Top with sliced onions and green pepper. Cook on "low" all day. Serve with spaghetti squash, top with shredded mozarella.

- Make a sausage stew as above but cut up the Italian sausages into quarters and add loads of mushrooms, celery, onions, and zucchini slices in with the sausage and tomato sauce. Serve with parmesan sprinkled over the stew.

For the Electric Skillet (think more one-dish meals):

- Pull out some boneless chicken breasts and saute in olive oil with garlic. Add sliced eggplant, zucchini, onions, green peppers, more olive oil, and cook until done. Salt and pepper and enjoy a skillet dinner in minutes.

- Saute beef fillets in oil. Replace top and cook through to desired doneness. Remove from skillet to plate. Now add more oil and saute sliced onions, green peppers and mushrooms. Top these on your beef. Steam assorted vegetables and dinner is served.

For the Pressure Cooker:
- Try Dr. Goldberg's favorite chicken soup recipe in the pressure cooker and create a classic dish in a fraction of the time.

- Make a stew in minutes.

- Buy the cheapest cuts of meat and make them taste like expensive cuts.

- Prepare a vegetable mushroom soup. Add cream just before serving.

This diet is great once you break out of your old eating patterns and move to really good, healthy foods. And don't think that you can't eat on the diet because of your ethnic heritage. Your ancestors and your family traditions aren't making you fat. It's a carbohy-drate- rich culture that causes your problems, not your grandparents! Let's get your imagination started.

Breakfasts

- Two large eggs scrambled in butter/olive oil mixture topped with one ounce of Swiss cheese; 1 cup of kefir, plain or artificially sweetened to taste

- Wheat bran waffles topped with strawberries; lean sausage; tea or coffee.

- Ricotta cheese pancakes; tea or coffee.

- Yogurt, artificially sweetened and mixed with chopped pecans and cinnamon; tea or coffee.

- Bacon and Eggs; high fiber crispbread with peanut butter; tea or coffee.

- Smoked fish, cheese slices, high fiber crispbread, and yogurt

- Fried steak and onions; high fiber crispbread; coffee.

- High fiber crispbreads with peanut butter or cream cheese-lox-tomato-capers and onions-; coffee or tea

- Chopped tomatoes, chopped cucumbers, and sprouts dressed with olive oil and tuna or smoked fish.

- String cheese, mixed nuts, coffee- on the run to the train.

Lunches

- Tuna salad made with real mayonnaise and pickle relish and hard boiled eggs.(Use one 6 oz. can of tuna per person); tossed salad with olive oil vinaigrette

- One can sardines packed in olive oil mashed with a hardboiled egg; cucumber slices; one ounce of macadamia or other nuts-and-seeds mix

- Deviled eggs, cheddar cheese and cucumber slices.

- Grilled chicken breast; multi-vegetable tossed salad with olive oil vinaigrette.

- Double cheeseburger (throw the bun in the garbage); tossed salad with olive oil vinaigrette.

- Cold roast chicken; broccoli salad with onions and cheese

- Egg salad; tossed salad with olive oil vinaigrette.

- Grilled or pan-fried or baked fish; steamed assorted vegetables

- Reheated leftovers from last-night's dinner.

- Two Polish or Italian sausages; sauerkraut; tossed salad

- Crustless Quiche, tossed salad with oil and vinegar; steamed vegetables

- Hearty Vegetable beef soup and tossed salad

Dinner

- Vegetable consommé; Roast chicken with mashed cauliflower; tossed salad with olive oil vinaigrette; small slice of artificially sweetened pumpkin pie made with a nut crust and served with whipped cream.

- Large steak, trimmed lean; fried onions; Stir-fried zucchini; tossed salad with olive oil vinaigrette; 1/2 cup strawberries and cream.

- Eggplant Parmesan ("bread" the eggplant with wheat bran and proceed with usual recipe); tossed salad with Olive oil vinaigrette; Blueberry and yogurt smoothie.

- Pork roast, acorn squash with butter and garlic, collard greens or creamed spinach; melon.

- Vegetable souffle; tossed salad with olive oil vinaigrette; sugar-free, flavored gelatin and whipped cream

- All beef hot dogs or bratwurst; sauerkraut; dill pickles; tossed salad with olive oil vinaigrette

- Chicken and vegetable stir fry on a bed of "riced" cauliflower; sugar-free cheesecake

- Meatballs and tomato sauce with spaghetti squash; tossed salad with olive oil vinaigrette; flavored coffee and real cream

- Deli meats and chopped liver; homemade coleslaw and pickles; Crispy lettuce leaves and crispbread to wrap meat.

- Pot roast with leeks, carrots, celery; mashed cauliflower; salad

- Grilled or baked fish; steamed broccoli and cauliflower; sautéed mushrooms

- Roasted Turkey; Grated zucchini and sausage stuffing; steamed vegetables; salad; Rhubarb crisp (topping made with ground nuts and bran) served with whipped cream

- Shishkabob with shrimp, scallops, chicken and vegetables; tossed salad with olive oil vinaigrette; Rootbeer float made with cream and diet rootbeer

- Grilled burgers, ribs, steaks, just about anything made on the grill provided you make your own barbeque sauce that is sweetened artificially. Try grilled vegetables seasoned with sugar free Italian dressing.

Snacks
- Nuts and seeds,

- kefir and yogurt smoothies,

- chicken wings roasted and dipped into a variety of no or low carbohydrate condiments,

- no-bake artificially sweetened cheesecakes, sugar-free pumpkin pie, strawberries, floats made from heavy cream and diet pop,

- hard salami slices and deli meats, cheese of all types, pork rinds,

- hardboiled and deviled eggs,

- fresh vegetables dipped in guacamole or salsa,

- high fiber crispbread with peanut butter or cream cheese or sour cream "chip" dips

- flavored coffees and cream.

By now, you probably have a good idea of how to create menus. You eat good food and make choices from the many, many low carbohydrate items that you are now getting accustomed to thinking about. Stretch your memory and try to think of home-cooking from your childhood. Many of those foods are on the diet! Like hearty, homemade soups and stews (just minus the potatoes and dumplings!).

Can you have a turkey dinner? Of course. Be sure to trim that roasted turkey with mashed cauliflower, asparagus and cheese sauce, mixed green salad, and baked acorn squash. Missing anything? Make a sugar-free pumpkin pie with whipped cream.

Can you make a breakfast on-the-run? Of course, pack up nuts and string cheese to eat on the train. Or maybe crispbread and peanut butter. Try a kefir shake.

It's getting easier, isn't it? We will give you recipes to get started with, but remember, you can adapt many of your favorite recipes too.

Chapter Eight: Recipes

In the next several pages, we will share a variety of recipes that have been prepared in our homes. The important point of this section is to get you thinking about creative ways to make low carbohydrate, high monounsaturated fat foods. Think about the food values. Plan to add fresh vegetables to all of your meal planning. Think about fiber and look for ways to add wheat bran or psyllium husks. Think about crushed nuts or high fiber crispbread as substitutes for graham cracker crusts.

Many of your favorite recipes can be made low carbohydrate by substituting no-calorie sweeteners for sugar and cream or kefir for milk. You can't use milled white or wheat flour, but you can use wheat bran, soy flour, and soy powder. It will take a lot of trial and error but it will pay off.

For instance, the famous canned pumpkin pie recipe can be on the diet by substituting granulated sugar substitute for sugar and cream or kefir for condensed milk. A ground nut crust can be made instead of the conventional piecrust. For a simple nut crust, coat a pie pan with spray canola oil, sprinkle ground nuts around the pan and tap the edge of the pan while turning it until the nuts coat the entire pan bottom and sides. Add your pie filling with the above modifications, bake and enjoy. The same crust can be made with wheat bran, too.

Can you think of other fillings? How about filling that crust with your favorite quiche recipe? It works perfectly on the diet! Quiche can also be made entirely "crustless". And, while we're speaking of eggs, souffles are on your diet now.

Your favorite cheesecake recipe is likewise adaptable to such substitutions. And a nut crust is far superior to graham crackers. Remember, except for the sugar in a cheesecake recipe, everything else is legal. So just take your favorite recipe, substitute a granulated no-calorie sugar substitute (this is really easy to find anywhere) and bake as usual.

There are many cookbooks on the market that can help you. For instance, vegetable and egg cookbooks will offer a variety of selections. Make sugar substitutions with no-calorie sweeteners when appropriate. There is even a brown sugar substitute.

The recipes we have included provide examples of how to calculate the carbohydrate and monounsaturated fat contents of your own recipes. Most meat, fish and egg recipes can be made low carbohydrate with little trouble. Look in French style cookbooks for sauces and foods that are usually low carbohydrate.

Use your imagination. For example, noodles are not allowed in soup. Substitute with finely shredded, lightly cooked, cabbage. Taco shells can be made from firm lettuce leaves. Or simply make a taco salad instead of tacos. Cauliflower can be cooked and mashed and used as a side dish like mashed potatoes or like a base for Chinese stir fry where you used to use rice or noodles. Spaghetti squash can be used in place of spaghetti and thinly sliced egglant can substitute for lasagna noodles in a meat and ricotta cheese or vegetable lasagna.

Wheat bran and ground nuts substitute for breadcrumbs for breading or as "fillers" in meatballs, meatloaf or even "stuffing". You can substitute grated zucchini, cauliflower or a mixture of both for potatoes in your recipe for latkes. And the real sour cream topping is allowed!

Don't panic. Many of your favorite recipes can be used "as is" without any changes. Especially soups, stews, and casseroles with cheeses and eggs. Watch out for corn, peas, beans, and potatoes in these recipes and either eliminate them or substitute an approved vegetable.

You still crave desserts? Well, what about artificially sweetened, flavored yogurts? Or "do-it-yourself" frozen yogurt. Or, diet flavored soda with 1-2 ounces of heavy cream or flavored coffees with a dollop of whipped cream.

Maybe, sugar free flavored gelatin and berries or high fiber crispbread and flavored cream cheese can satisfy the dessert urge. Or artificially sweetened chopped rhubarb with a crisp crust of crushed nuts, bran, artificial brown sugar and butter "crisped" in the oven. Energetic? Make a dessert souffle with granulated sugar substitute. Too pooped? Make a package of instant, sugar-free pudding mixed with kefir instead of milk.

Get involved. Very soon you will be eating to live, not living to eat. And you won't miss the garbage you had been eating.

A few inexpensive kitchen gadgets make life much easier.
- A waffle iron.

- A yogurt incubator.

- A good blender with a heavy duty motor. Making smoothies and cheesecakes and pumpkin pies is so easy when your blender can handle the task.

- A pressure cooker

- A crockpot

- An electric skillet

- An ice cream maker (Yes, it's allowed if you make it with real cream or if you make your own frozen yogurt)

Get involved with the diet. Read as much as you can. Try recipes. Make the commitment. For those who have internet capabilities, do a search on low carbohydrate dieting. Join newsgroups. Make friends with others who are your kindred spirits in this endeavor. Most of all, good luck with your diet.

Note: Many of the names used are registered trademarks of their manufacturers.
Nutrasweet is a registered trademark of the Nutrasweet Company
Sweet N' Low is a registered trademark of Cumberland Packing Corp.
SweetOne as a registered trademark of Stadt Corporation
Sunette is a registered trademark of Hoechst AG.
Sugar Twin is a registered trademark of Alberto Culver, USA, Inc.
Sweet-10 is a registered trademark of The Pilsbury Co.
Metamucil is a registered trademark of Proctor and Gamble

Goldberg-O'Mara Diet
Recipe for: LowCarb Breads
Category: Breads, Cakes, Cookies   Serves 6

Amt.	Measure	Ingredient	Fat	Mono%	Carb	Protein
1/4	Cup	Soda water (Seltzer)				
1/4	Teaspoon	Salt				
4	Tablespoons	Mayonnaise	10	60	0	2
4	Large	Eggs	20	39	2	25
1/4	Cup	soy or whey protein	0		0	24
1/2	Cup	Wheat bran	1		6	4
1	Packet	Sweetener				
		Totals	31	40	8	55
		Per Serving	**5**	**40**	**1**	**9**

Instructions: Combine eggs water and mayonnaise in a blender. You can beat by hand with a whisk, but the blender gives a finer grain to the bread. Blend 30 seconds. Add in soy or whey protein and wheat bran. Bake in greased 8" loaf pan at 375°F for about 35 minutes.

Variations:

A sweet bread can be made increasing the sweetener, adding nutmeg, vanilla, cinnamon, cloves etc. When baked brush the loaf with melted butter and sprinkle sweetener and cinnamon over top.

For a banana bread add banana flavoring and walnuts. Sprinkle sweetener and ground cinnamon over top when baked.

Goldberg-O'Mara Diet
Recipe for: Muffins
Category: Breads, Cakes, Cookies   Makes 12

Amt.	Measure	Ingredient	Fat	Mono%	Carb	Protein
1/2	Cup	Soy or whey protein	0		0	48
1/2	Cup	Wheat bran	1		6	4
1/2	Cup	Soda Water	0	0	10	2
4	Large	Eggs	20	39	2.5	17
1/2	teaspoon	cinnamon				
1/4	teaspoon	ground nutmeg				
1	teaspoon	Vanilla Extract				
1/4	Cup	Cream	11	28	1	0.5
3	Packets	Sugar Twin			4	
3	Packets	Sweet-One			3	
		Totals	32	36	26	72
		Per Muffin	**3**	**36**	**2**	**6**

Instructions: Preheat oven to 400°F. Place the eggs, cream, water, nutmeg, extracts, and sweetener in a blender . Add in soy or whey protein and the wheat bran mixture then blend till smooth. The batter is very thin. Grease 12 muffin cups or use paper or foil liners.

Divide batter into tins. Bake 20 min. or until done. Eat with a thick pat of butter or cream cheese.

Great source of soy protein with the heart protection of the phytoestrogens.

Remember to use Soy protein and not soy flour.

Goldberg-O'Mara Diet
Recipe for: Almond Macaroons
Category: Breads, Cakes, Cookies   Makes 24

Amt.	Measure	Ingredient	Fat	Mono%	Carb	Protein
4	each	Egg whites	0	0	1	13
1	teaspoon	Almond Flavor				
1	teaspoon	Vanilla				
1_	cups	Ground almonds	50	62	12	20
6	packets	SweetOne (Sunette)			6	
6	packets	Sugar Twin			6	
		Totals	50	62	25	33
		Per Cookie	**2**	**62**	**1**	**1.3**

Instructions: Beat eggwhites stiff but not dry. Add almond and vanilla flavorings at the end of the beating. Mix the sweeteners and the nuts together, then fold in the egg whites.

Drop by teaspoon onto baking sheets. Bake at 350°F for 20 minutes.

When cooled, store in an air-tight plastic bag or container.

Goldberg-O'Mara Diet
Recipe for: Coconut and Almond Macaroons
Category: Breads, Cakes, Cookies   Makes 24

Amt.	Measure	Ingredient	Fat	Mono%	Carb	Protein
4	each	egg whites	0	0	1	13
1/2	teaspoon	coconut flavor				
1	teaspoon	vanilla				
1/2	Cup	chopped almonds or pecans	16	62	4	6.5
1	Cup	dried ground coconut plus_ water	64	33	8	7
6	Packets	SweetOne (Sunette)			6	
6	Packets	Sugar Twin			6	
		Totals	80	40	25	26.5
		Per Cookie	**3.5**	**40**	**1**	**1.1**

Instructions: Beat eggwhites stiff but not dry. Add almond and coconut flavorings at the end of the beating. Mix the other ingredients then fold in the egg mixture. Drop by teaspoon onto baking sheets. Bake at 350°F for 20 minutes. When cooled, store in an airtight plastic bag or container.

Goldberg-O'Mara Diet
Recipe for: NoBake Chocolate Cheesecake
Category: Breads, Cakes, Cookies   Servings 10

Amt.	Measure	Ingredient	Fat	Mono%	Carb	Protein
1	package	gelatin	0	0	0	6
1	teaspoon	Vanilla	0	0	0	0
1	cup	boiling water	0	0	0	0
16	Ounce	cream cheese, softened	157	29	12	33
18	Packets	Equal or Sunnette SweetOne	0	0	18	0
2	Ounce	Unsweetened baking chocolate			6	
		Totals	157	29	36	39
		Per Serving	**16**	**29**	**3.6**	**4**

Instructions: Melt the chocolate in a double boiler or just microwave it with the cream cheese. Dissolve the gelatin in the boiling water in a mixing bowl. Combine all the ingredients and stir well. Beat well with an electric mixer or place in a blender for a minute or until smooth.. Pour into prepared muffin cups. Place the muffin tray in the refrigerator and chill until firm, about 2 hours. (Makes 10)

Goldberg-O'Mara Diet
Recipe for: Broccoli Soup
Category: Soups Serves 1

Amt.	Measure	Ingredient	Fat	Mono%	Carb	Protein
1	cup	Chicken stock or water				
1	oz	cream cheese	9	29	0.9	7
1/4	cup	sharp cheddar cheese	11	29	0.4	8.3
2	tablespoon	heavy cream	9	28	0.7	0.5
1	cup	chopped broccoli	0	0	3.5	3.6
1/4	teaspoon	Cumin powder				
		Totals	**29**	**29**	**5.5**	**19.4**

Instructions: Steam the broccoli until tender. Add the tender broccoli to the cheeses, broth and cumin in a blender or use a hand blender. Salt and pepper to taste. Bring to a boil to melt the cheese. Serve piping hot and adding the cream at the table. A sprinkle of grated parmesan or romano cheese completes the dish.

This is a recipe for one large serving. Served with a tossed salad dressed with an olive oil and vinegar will balance out the monounsaturated fats. and it makes a satisfying lunch.

Goldberg-O'Mara Diet
Recipe for: Chocolates
Category: Get me through the evening medicine
Makes 64 squares in a 8x8 pan

Amt.	Measure	Ingredient	Fat	Mono%	Carb	Protein
3	ounces	Cocoa butter	84		0	
2	Tablespoons	cocoa			4	
8	ounces	Cream cheese	79	29	6	17
3	Tablespoon	butter	40	28	0	
4	Tablespoon	heavy cream	16	28	1	
1/2	Teaspoon	vanilla extract			1	
14	Packets	Nutrasweet or Sweet-one			14	
4	Tablespoon	chopped walnuts, Macadamias or Chunky Peanut butter	28	50	12	
		Totals	247		38	
		Per chocolate	**4**	**29**	**1**	

Instructions: Melt the cocoa butter, butter and cream cheese together in a bowl over boiling water. (or microwave for about 2 minutes.) Stir in the cocoa.

Using a rubber spatula, mix in the the cream, vanilla and nuts. Stir until smooth. When cool add the sweetener. (You may want additional sweetener if it is too bitter for you)

Drop onto parchment paper and refrigerate for at least two hours (much better overnight).

Alternatively, pour the mixture onto a nonstick cookie sheet and refrigerate. Cut into squares then store refrigerated.

Dosage. Take one or two when you get the urge.

Goldberg-O'Mara Diet
Recipe for: Eggplant Lasagna
Category: Main Course   8 servings

Amt.	Measure	Ingredient	Fat	Mono%	Carb	Protein
8	tablespoon	Olive oil	110	74	0	0
1	teaspoon	Oregano	0	0	0	0
1	teaspoon	Basil	0	0	0	0
2	teaspoon	Garlic powder			4	
1	teaspoon	Onion powder			2	
		pepper and salt to taste	0	0	0	0
1	large	Eggplant sliced 1/2-in thick	0	0	11	3
8	ounce	Mozzarella cheese sliced	45	29	4.5	40
2	large	Eggs	10	39	2	8.5
2	14 ounce can	Stewed tomatoes	0	0	10	2
1	large	Onion			10	2
1	cup	Freshly grated Parmesan	30	29	3.8	42
1	cup	Wheat bran	3		12	9
		Totals	198	50	60	106
		Per Serving	**25**	**50**	**8**	**13**

Instructions: To make the sauce, finely chop the onion and sauté in about 6 tablespoons of the oil until translucent. Add the oregano, basil, salt and pepper and tomatoes with the liquid from the can and 1 teaspoon of the garlic powder. Beat one egg with one tablespoon of water, salt, pepper, onion powder, and garlic powder. Dip the eggplant slices in the egg mixture them coat with the wheatbran. Lay the eggplant slices in a single layer on a baking sheet and brush them with oil.. Broil them close to the heat for 5 minutes or until cooked. Turn, brush the other side with the oil, and broil until the second side is done.

Instructions, *continued*

Preheat oven to 350°F. Make a layer with half the eggplant slices in a wide, shallow baking dish. Add half the tomato sauce, then layer in half of the mozzarella, and Parmesan. Repeat the layering with the second half of the ingredients. Bake 20-to-25 minutes or until hot and bubbly. Allow to cool for about 10 minutes before cutting. This dish makes excellent leftovers for lunch.

Goldberg-O'Mara Diet
Recipe for: Mayonnaise
Category: Sauces   Makes 24 tablespoons

Amt.	Measure	Ingredient	Fat	Mono%	Carb	Protein
2	large	egg yolks	10	39	1	6
2	tablespoon	lemon juice	0	0	0	0
2	tablespoon	water	0	0	0	0
1	packet	sugar substitute	0	0	1	0
1	teaspoon	dry mustard	0	0	0	0
1	pinch	salt	0	0	0	0
	dash	pepper	0	0	0	0
1	cup	light olive oil or Canola oil	216	74	0	0
		Totals	226	73	2	6
		Per Tablespoon	**10**	**73**	**0.2**	**0.25**

Instructions: This recipe cooks the yolks for safety. In small saucepan, stir all the ingredients except the oil until thoroughly blended. Cook over very low heat, stirring constantly, until mixture just starts to boil. Remove from heat. Let stand a few minutes to cool. Pour into blender container. Cover and blend at high speed. While blending, very slowly add oil. Blend until thick and smooth. Occasionally, turn off blender and scrape down sides of container with rubber spatula. Cover and chill if not using immediately.

Keeps refrigerated about one week. Use the left over egg whites for the cookie recipes.

Goldberg-O'Mara Diet
Recipe for: Alfredo Sauce
Category: Sauces   Makes 37 tablespoon servings

Amt.	Measure	Ingredient	Fat	Mono%	Carb	Protein
2	Cups	Heavy cream	88	28	7	5
1	Large	Egg	5	39	1	6
1	Tablespoon	Crushed garlic			3	
1/4	Teaspoon	Black Pepper				
1/3	Cup	Fresh grated parmesan cheese	7.5	29	1	11
3	Tablespoon	Unsalted butter	35	28		
		Totals	135		12	22
		Per tablespoon	**3.6**	**29**	**0.3**	**1**

Instructions: Pour cream into a heavy saucepan, add the butter, and heat until warm on a low heat.

Beat egg lightly with a fork and add to the pan. Add the pepper and garlic. Start whisking the mixture when butter has melted. When the sauce is hot slowly add the cheese. Raise the heat until almost boiling. Keep whisking until the sauce is smooth. Remove the pot from the heat and serve the hot sauce over vegetables, eggs or anything else you want. Note: This has a low percentage of monounsaturated fat. Eat a salad with olive oil vinaigrette to balance.

Goldberg-O'Mara Diet
Recipe for: Caesar's Dressing
Category: Sauces   Makes 14 Tablespoons

Amt.	Measure	Ingredient	Fat	Mono%	Carb	Protein
1/3	Cup	Mayonnaise (homemade)	50	75		
1/4	Cup	Finely grated parmesean cheese	7.5	29	1	10.5
2	tablespoon	Fresh squeezed lemon or lime juice			2	
2	tablespoon	Water				
8	each	Anchovies chopped fine	1.5	40	0	4.5
1/2	teaspoon	Freshly ground pepper				
1/4	teaspoon	minced garlic or garlic powder				
		Totals	59	70	3	1.5
		Per Tablespoon	**4**	**70**	**0.2**	**1**

Instructions: Crush the anchovies with the back of a spoon against a small bowl then blend all ingredients together. If it gets too thick just add a little water to thin it out.

Goldberg-O'Mara Diet
Recipe for: Pancake or Waffle
Category: Breakfast   Serves 1

Amt.	Measure	Ingredient	Fat	Mono%	Carb	Protein
1	Large	Egg	5	39	1	6
1/3	Cup	Wheat Bran	1		4	3
1/2	Teaspoon	Psyllium Powder (Metamucil)				
1/4	Cup	Nut flour (optional)	8	62	2	3
1/4	Teaspoon	Flavoring e.g. Vanilla Extract				
1	Packet	Sugar Twin or SweetOne Sunette			1	
1/2	Cup	Water				
1/4	Teaspoon	Baking powder (leave out for waffle)				
1	Tablespoon	Olive oil for frying	13	75		
	TOPPING					
1/2	Cup	Plain yogurt or kefir	4	30	2	4
1	Packet	Nutrasweet			1	
		Totals	31	59	11	16

Instructions: Combine all ingredients and beat with a fork until smooth. Heat an omelet pan and add the olive oil. (Medium to low heat or the pancake will burn). Add the pancake mix and fry for about 2 minutes. Turn with a spatula and cook for a further two minutes. (To make into a waffle, add the oil to the batter then add to the waffle iron.)

While frying, wash your bowl and add the yogurt or Kefir. Add the packet of nutrasweet or use liquid saccharine. Stir with a fork to mix. To flavor the topping, you may want to add a few drops of maple extract or vanilla extract. To eat, take a bite-sized piece of pancake or waffle and dip it into the sweetened yogurt, then pop it straight to your mouth.

This is a very satisfying breakfast pancake. It supplies most of your daily fiber needs for regularity. It is also satisfying and keeps you going until lunch.

Other topping suggestions. Sour Cream, 1 strawberry mashed with 2 tablespoons of water then sweetened to taste.

Note: You can make this in a big batch and freeze the individual pancakes or waffles in a plastic sandwich bag. Microwave for three minutes for a quick breakfast.

Goldberg-O'Mara Diet
Recipe for: Peanut Butter Ice Cream
Category: Dessert   Six servings

Amt.	Measure	Ingredient	Fat	Mono%	Carb	Protein
6	Large	Eggs separated	32	39	3.3	38
1	teaspoon	Vanilla				
6	packets	sugar substitute			3	
3	tablespoons	chunky peanut butter	50	24	15	25
1/2	pint	heavy cream	90	28	6	5
		Totals	172	28	27	68
		Per Cookie	**29**	**28**	**4.5**	**11**

Instructions: Beat egg yolks, vanilla and 3 packets of sugar substitute until light in color.

Stir in peanut butter until smooth. Whip the cream with remaining sugar substitute. Fold whipped cream into peanut butter mixture. Beat egg whites until stiff peaks form and fold into mixture. Pour into freezer trays or individual serving cups. Cover with transparent wrap and freeze until firm. If ice cream has been in the freezer for more than six hours allow to stand at room temp 15 minutes before serving.

Goldberg-O'Mara Diet
Recipe for: Pumpkin Pie
Category: Dessert   Serves 8

Amt.	Measure	Ingredient	Fat	Mono%	Carb	Protein
1	15 oz Can	Libby's Pumpkin	2		14	7
3	Large	Eggs	15	39	2	19
1 1/2	Cups	Water				
1	Teaspoon	Cinnamon			2	
1/2	Teaspoon	Ginger			1	
2	Oz	Crushed or ground Almonds	30	65	10	11
1	Teaspoon	Vanilla Extract				
1/2	Teaspoon	Almond Extract				
1	Tablespoon	Olive oil	13.5	74		
8	Packets	Sugar Twin	0	0	8	0
8	Packets	Sweet-One (Sunette)	0	0	8	0
		Totals	60.5	62	45	37
		Per Slice	**7.5**	**62**	**5.5**	**4.4**

Instructions: Oil a 9 inch pie dish (pyrex) and sprinkle with crushed or powdered nuts to make a crust. Blend all remaining ingredients in a blender. (Do not use Nutrasweet® since it breaks down with high heat) Pour mixture over nuts. Bake at 425 °F for 15 minutes then bake at 350°F for 35-40 minutes.Cool, then refrigerate.

Makes 8 servings. Top with whipped cream sweetened with artificial sweeteners.

Goldberg-O'Mara Diet
Recipe for: Basic Quiche
Category: Main Course or breakfast Serves 4

Amt.	Measure	Ingredient	Fat	Mono%	Carb	Protein
3	Large	Eggs	15	39	2	19
1	Cup	heavy cream	90	28	7	5
1	Cup	grated cheddar cheese	33	29	1	25
		Additions of choice*				
		Pepper to taste				
		Totals	138	30	10	49
		Per Serving	**35**	**30**	**3**	**10**

Instructions: Combine all with a whisk. Pour into quiche or pie plate and bake at 350°F for 45 minutes.

*ADDITIONS: You can add bacon, green onions and Swiss cheese to make a traditional quiche Lorraine, sausage, peppers, onions, mozzarella, spinach, Swiss or feta cheese, onions, and salsa. Serve topped with sour cream.

Makes a fantastic quiche with leftover vegetables such as cauliflower, broccoli etc.

Be creative!!!!!

To balance the fats, eat with a tossed salad with olive oil/ vinegar dressing.

Goldberg-O'Mara Diet
Recipe for: Vegetable Quiche
Category: Entree or Breakfast Serves 6

Amt.	Measure	Ingredient	Fat	Mono%	Carb	Protein
2	Cups	Cooked Cauliflower	1		4	4
1	Cup	Grated cheddar Cheese	37	30	1.5	28
4	Large	Eggs	20	39	3	25
1	Cup	Cream or half and half	44	30	3.3	2
1	Teaspoon	Salt				
		Pepper to taste				
1	Tablespoon	Olive oil to grease pan	13	75		
		Totals	115	37	12	59
		Per portion	**19**	**37**	**2**	**10**

Instructions: Blend all the ingredients reserving about 1/4 cup of the cheese and the oil.

Oil a casserole dish or a 9 inch pyrex pie dish with the oil. Pour in the blended mixture.

Sprinkle the top with the remaining cheese. Bake in a 350 °F oven for 40 minute. Let cool for about 10 minutes to set before eating. Makes 8 portions.

Fantastic Sunday lunch eaten with a tossed green salad. Use Olive oil and vinegar dressing to balance the monounsaturated fats. Portions freeze well.

Goldberg-O'Mara Diet
Recipe for: Ricotta Pancakes
Category: Main or Breakfast

Amt.	Measure	Ingredient	Fat	Mono%	Carb	Protein
8	ounces	ricotta cheese	27	29	6	22
1	tablespoon	olive oil	13	74	0	0
1/2	Cup	almond powder	28	65.5	3.5	10
2	large	Eggs	10	39	1	12.5
1	package	Sunette Sweet One	0	0	1	0
1	teaspoon	Vanilla	0	0	0	0
1	pinch	Salt	0	0	0	0
3	tablespoon	Oil - for frying	39	74	0	0
		Totals	117	56	11.5	44.5

Instructions: Mix all ingredients until you make a smooth batter. Add one tablespoon of oil to a crepe pan. And heat to moderately hot. Add a few tablespoons of batter into pan. Swirl the pan to spread the batter. They form very thin pancakes like crepes or blintzes. Cook on first side until bubbly and brown around edges. Let firm up before turning.

Turn gently and fry until done.

Goldberg-O'Mara Diet
Recipe for: Salmon Patties
Category: Main Course

Amt.	Measure	Ingredient	Fat	Mono%	Carb	Protein
1	can	Red Salmon (Use the bones too)	27	38	0	75
2	Large	Eggs	10	39	0	12.5
1/2	Cup	Chopped onion	0.1		3	0.5
1/4	Cup	Chopped red or yellow pepper	0	0	1.5	0.2
1	Stalk	Chopped celery	0	0	1	0.2
2	Tablespoons	Wheat bran	0.2		1	0.6
1/4	Cup	Olive oil for frying	54	74	0	0
1/2	Teaspoon	Salt	0	0	0	0
		Totals	**91.3**	**59**	**6.5**	**89**
		PER PATTY	9.1	59	0.65	8.9
	TARTAR	SAUCE				
4	Tablespoon	Real mayonnaise	40	73	1	1
2	Tablespoon	Dill relish	0	0	1	1

Instructions: Mash all the ingredients together. Form patties (makes 8 - 10 patties) Fry in the oil about 2 - 3 minutes each side. Serve with the tartar sauce and a tossed salad.

Goldberg-O'Mara Diet
Recipe for: Spinach Pie
Category: Main Course   **Serves 6**

Amt.	Measure	Ingredient	Fat	Mono%	Carb	Protein
3	Tablespoon	Olive oil	40	74	0	0
1	Medium	Onion–chopped	0	0	10	2
10	ounces	Frozen chopped Spinach–thawed, Squeezed	0	0	2	9
1/2	Teaspoon	Salt	0	0	0	0
1/2	Teaspoon	Pepper	0	0	0	0
1/4	Teaspoon	Ground nutmeg	0	0	0	0
15	ounces	Ricotta cheese	32	29	8	30
8	ounces	Mozzarella cheese–grated	50	29	5	45
1	Cup	Parmesan cheese–grated	30	29	4	42
3	large	Eggs–beaten	15	39	2	13
1		Frozen pie crust				
		Totals	**167**	**42**	**31**	**31**
		Per portion	28	42	5	5

Instructions: Preheat oven to 350°F. Melt butter in heavy large skillet over medium heat. Add onion and sauté until tender, about 8 minutes. Mix in spinach, salt, pepper and nutmeg. Sauté until all liquid from spinach evaporates, about 3 minutes.

Combine ricotta, mozzarella and Parmesan cheeses in large bowl. Mix in eggs.

Add spinach mixture; blend well. Spoon cheese mixture into pie crust. Bake until filling is set in center and brown on top, about 40 minutes. Let stand 10 minutes. Cut pie into 6 pieces. You can feed the pie to the family, but you must not eat your portion of the crust.

Eat with a small tossed salad with olive oil and vinegar dressing to balance the fats.

Goldberg-O'Mara Diet
Recipe for: Mashed Potatoes Substitute
Category: Vegetable   Serves 6

Amt.	Measure	Ingredient	Fat	Mono%	Carb	Protein
4	Cups	Chopped cauliflower			8	8
2	tablespoons	Dried minced onions			6	1
1	Cup	Mayonnaise	160	73	1	4
2	each	Eggs	10	39	2	8
		Salt and pepper to taste				
		Totals	170	70	17	21
		Per Serving	28		3	3.5

Instructions: Hard boil the eggs and cool. Boil the cauliflower until overdone and soggy. Drain, mix in the onion powder and let cool for ten minutes. Add the eggs, mayonnaise, some salt and pepper and mash all together. Salt and pepper to taste.

Goldberg-O'Mara Diet
Recipe for: Zucchini Latkes
Category: Side dish.   Serves 6

Amt.	Measure	Ingredient	Fat	Mono%	Carb	Protein
8	small	Zucchini (peel if skin is bitter)			16	12
1	large	Onion			10	2
1/3	Cup	Soy flour	6	22	10	10
3	large	Eggs	15	38	2	19
1	teaspoon	Baking powder				
1	Cup	Canola oil	216	73		
1/4	teaspoon	Pepper				
1	teaspoon	Salt				
1	packet	Sweet n' low			1	1
		Totals	236	72	39	44
		Per Serving	39	72	6.5	7

Instructions: Grate the onion and zucchini together Add the salt and allow to drain for about 10 minutes in a colander. Squeeze the excess moisture out. Add the eggs, pepper, baking powder, sweetener and soy flour. Mix well. Preheat heavy pan filled with the oil to a depth of about 1/4 inch. Drop tablespoonfuls into hot oil. Fry on medium heat for about one to two minutes. Turn over and continue to fry until well browned. Drain the pancakes on a paper towel and serve hot. Serve with sour cream, yogurt or kefir. Makes about 4 latkes per person.

Goldberg-O'Mara Diet
Recipe for: Kefir Smoothie
Category: Snack   Serves 1

Amt.	Measure	Ingredient	Fat	Mono%	Carb	Protein
1/2	Cup	Plain Kefir			2	
1/2	Cup	Blueberries or Strawberries			5	
1/2	Cup	Ice cubes				
1	Packet	Nutrasweet or Sweet n'low			1	
		Totals			8	

Instructions: Place all ingredients in a blender and blend until smooth. You may need to add a tablespoon of water if it gets too thick. Pour into a tall glass and sip through a straw.

Goldberg-O'Mara Diet
Recipe for: Kefir or Yogurt
Category: Dairy

Amt.	Measure	Ingredient	Fat	Mono%	Carb	Protein
1	Quart	Whole milk			*	
1	Ounce	Starter				

* Two thirds of the milk carbohydrates will be removed by the culture.

Instructions: You will need to purchase your first live culture kefir or yogurt from the grocery store. Buy only the plain kefir or yogurt with no fruit or sugar added. You can eat it all except for the first liquid ounce which you will use as a starter for your next batch.

Place the bottle of milk into a large pot containing enough water to cover half the bottle. If you by milk in a carton, transfer it to a clean glass bottle. Open the lid a little to allow for expansion of the liquid and air. Bring the water to a boil. And simmer for about 5 minutes. You have now pasteurized your milk. Allow the pasteurized milk to cool to room temperature. Add your one ounce (about two tablespoons) of kefir or yogurt starter to the each quart of cooled milk and put the bottle cap on. Mix the starter with the milk. Place the bottle on the top of your refrigerator and leave it there for at least 24 hours. In cool climates you may need 36 to 48 hours. Congratulations. You have just made a quart of kefir or yogurt. Use all of it except for the last ounce which you will use as the starter for your next batch.

The homemade kefir or yogurt will keep very well for up to two weeks in the refrigerator. In fact, the Kefir becomes smooth and creamy after about a week in the refrigerator and the yogurt flavor improves.

To eat the kefir or yogurt, pour or spoon about half a cup into a cup or bowl. Add sweetener and flavorings (such as coconut and pineapple extracts if you want a pina colada flavor). Beat the mixture with a fork for about 30 seconds and you will have a thick creamy liquid which you can drink or use as a topping for pancakes.

Goldberg-O'Mara Diet
Recipe for: Cold Float
Category: Drink

Amt.	Measure	Ingredient	Fat	Mono%	Carb	Protein
2	Tablespoon	Heavy cream			1	
1	glass	Carbonated Diet Beverage			0	
		Total			1	

Instructions: You can add a couple of tablespoons of cream to any carbonated drink to make a creamy float. Tastes fantastic with root beer or diet chocolate fudge..

Goldberg-O'Mara Diet
Recipe for: Cheese Omelet
Category: Breakfast   One serving

Amt.	Measure	Ingredient	Fat	Mono%	Carb	Protein
2	Large	Eggs	10	39	2	8
2	Tablespoon	Heavy cream	11	29	1	1
1/4	Teaspoon	salt				
1/4	Cup	Grated cheddar or Swiss cheese	8	29	1	9
1	Tablespoon	Sweet butter	13	29		
1	Tablespoon	Olive oil	13	74		
		Total	55	38	4	18

Instructions: A good omelet pan is essential. If you don't have one, you can still use a frying pan, but the right tool for the job is such a help. Beat together the eggs, cream and salt. Heat the pan and melt the butter. Add the oil. Lower the heat to medium and add the egg mixture. Using a spatula, keep pushing the edge of the egg mixture towards the center of the pan allowing the liquid center egg to flow back out. Work your way around the pan. When almost cooked, sprinkle the cheese over one half of the pan. Ease the omelet onto a plate. When half way out of the pan fold the omelet over onto itself. Enjoy.

Many other fillings can be used. Raw chopped vegetable, sautéed vegetables, smoked salmon for a savory omelet.

Some More Recipes and Suggestions

We have now gone through a number of recipes and have shown you how to calculate the contribution of carbohydrates and fats from the individual ingredients. You're probably pretty good by now. Most of the time, we're rushing through life and do not have time to cook. Here are a few last minute suggestions for our hectic lives.

Recipe for Salads

Remember to make lots of salads with fresh garden vegetables like leaf lettuce, arugala, spinach, sliced onions, tomatoes, cucumbers, peppers and all the wonderful bounty of low carbohydrate vegetables. Mix in sliced hard-boiled eggs, sliced ham, turkey, cold boiled chicken, bacon bits, cheese cubes or anything else that is low in carbohydrates.

Recipe for Ratatouille

Cube one large eggplant and two medium zucchini squash. Slice up one medium onion , one red pepper and one green pepper. Add 1/4 cup of olive oil to a large skillet and saute several cloves if sliced garlic. Over medium heat add the cubed eggplant and zucchini. Add the peppers and onions. Sprinkle with thyme, basil and oregano to taste. Add salt and pepper to taste. Cook until the eggplant is soft and brown in color adding more oil as needed. Dice the tomatoes from one can of Italian plum tomatoes and add to the pot. Cook for another 5 minutes then serve hot or cold as a side dish.

Recipe for : Upside-down Pizza

Coat a glass ovenproof casserole dish with canola oil. Build an upside down pizza as follows:
Bottom layer : Sliced Italian sausage or pepperoni
Next layer: Sliced mushrooms, chopped spinach, sliced onions, peppers and other toppings. Next layer: one can diced canned tomatoes or fresh tomato slices. Next layer: Sprinkle with oregano, crushed garlic and crushed red peppers to taste. Finally top with a generous layer of mozarella or mixed shredded pizza cheeses.
Bake at 400 F until top melts and browns. Serve straight from the dish.

Recipe for Smoked Salmon Cheese Spread

Blend together a one pound can of salmon with one pound of cream cheese. Add some finely chopped onions. Add one teaspoon of liquid smoke and salt and pepper to taste. Blend with a large fork or spoon until smooth. Serve with celery sticks, cucumber slices or Fiber Rye Crackers. Yummy for a party.

Dr. Goldberg's Chicken Soup.

Coarsely chop three celery sticks, one medium carrot, a small bunch of parsley and 10 okra. Wash and cut up a three pound chicken. Remove the skin from the backs, thighs and breast. Place everything in a 6-quart pressure cooker. Add one tablespoon of salt and 1 teaspoon of pepper. Add water to fill the pot no more than two thirds full. Close the lid. Place on high heat until full pressure according to the instructions for your pot. Lower the heat and cook at full pressure for 20 minutes. Remove the pot from the heat and allow it to cool until the pressure has fallen.

Open the pot and remove the chicken, which can be eaten as the main course or made into a salad or patties when cold. Serve the soup with the vegetables and finely shredded, slightly cooked green cabbage as a "noodle" supplement.

Summary

In the summer, remember to grill meats and fish on the backyard grill. Keep cole slaw or broccoli slaw in the refrigerator for side dishes. Slice vegetables and marinade in seasoned oil and vinegar or lemon, then throw these on the grill, too. Dress chopped onions, green peppers, and tomatoes with oil and vinegar, salt and pepper and keep in a covered container in the refrigerator for a healthy side salad. Be creative with vegetables. Construct a bacon-lettuce-and tomato salad.

In cold weather, use that crockpot and make pot roast, chili, and stews. For chili, use only one can of kidney beans to a full pot of chili so that the carbohydrate count will be low per serving size. Add celery for more texture and fiber. Top with chopped onions, green pepper, shredded cheese, and guacamole. Put a small pot roast or boneless pork roast in the crockpot, cover with salsa, and cook on low all day. When you get home, shred the meat and turn it into a taco salad by putting the meat on a bed of lettuce and topping it with sour cream, guacamole, cheese, and salsa.

Have fun with this diet. You are now eating much more nutritiously and in the process, losing weight. You will never need to go back to the unhealthy eating habits that only created problems for you. We've all learned something in this journey and with open minds, we'll learn a lot more in the future. Good health to you from both of us!

Chapter Nine:
Help! I'm not losing weight.

"Why am I not losing weight? I've followed the diet faithfully and I can't seem to lose. I think I've hit a plateau. Maybe, this won't work for me."

We've heard this more than once. After a brisk 4-pound weight loss in the first week, people are upset when they go the next week with no change in the scale. Is this a diet failure? Or they lose 12 pounds in the first month and then can't seem to move the scale at all for three weeks. Is this a sign of failure? Or they have a nice 1-2 pound weight loss every week for three months then mysteriously stop when they still have several pounds to go. Is this usual? No, there are many reasons for the start-and-stop behavior on the diet.

First of all, plateaus are common. You didn't put on the weight evenly and non stop and you won't take it off evenly and non-stop. These plateaus are your body catching its breath. Sometimes they last a week, sometimes a month. Don't' let these little bumps throw you off the straight and narrow path to a slimmer you. Relax and let your body take you there. It WILL happen.

One of the worst things you can do while dieting (and of course we ALL do it) is to weigh ourselves at every opportunity, whenever we're near that bathroom scale. Isn't it amazing that your weight can vary so much over the course of the day? But changes over the day reflect changes in water more than fat. The best reflection of fat loss is your waist measurement. That doesn't change minute-to-minute.

Women sometimes hold onto water at various times of the month. A rapid change in weight day to day is just water retention and loss. It takes about 3500 calories to gain or lose a pound of fat. So a three-pound loss in one day is usually just a water shift because you certainly cannot burn off 10,500 calories in one day unless you're running a marathon!

A common reason for a slow weight loss is a drug interference. Many drugs act on the stress hormones which counteract the mechanisms we are trying to induce with the Goldberg-O'Mara diet. Steroid drugs are the biggest culprits followed by non-steroidal anti-inflammatory drugs including asprin and ibuprofen, estrogens such as birth control pills and hormone replacement therapies, blood pressure medications and antidepressants. **Do not stop any drug without your physician's guidance.** You have been given these drugs for a medical reason and you should follow your physician's advice. The diet may still work for you, just at a slower rate. So please be patient.

A sluggish thyroid gland can slow things down. If you have not been tested for hypothyroidism in the past year, ask your doctor to check this out with a blood test named Thyroid Stimulating Hormone often shortened to "TSH". Sometimes, a perfectly normal thyroid gland can become sluggish because of a lack of iodine in the diet. We suggest you always use iodized salt to maintain a plentiful supply of iodine.

Not eating enough can also slow weight loss to a crawl. Believe it! If your body senses that its not getting enough calories, it SLOWS your metabolism to compensate. It thinks it's starving so it will try to preserve calories by slowing all systems down. DO NOT skip meals or try to reduce calories to try to speed up your weight loss. It just won't work long term. It actually works against you.

Hidden carbohydrates are another weight loss trap. You think you're eating less than 40 grams per day, but you forgot to count the 1 gram per packet of sweetener and you use 10 packets per day. Don't forget to look at ALL labels and COUNT every source of carbohydrates. Don't trust food labels alone. Make sure they agree with your carbohydrate counter book. Always assume the worst case.

Some food sensitivities can affect some people. Examples are caffeine, citric acid in soft drinks, nuts, dairy products like cheese, or red meat. Different strokes for different folks. Try cutting certain foods out of your diet to see if it helps.

And finally, alas there are a few individuals who will not lose by this diet. We don't know why. Maybe we missed something in counting the carbohydrates. Maybe the hyperinsulinemia is not easily shut off and even our reduced carbohydrate limits are too high and end up processed into fat stores. However, don't think you are one of these people until you've given the diet a truly fair chance of about 6 months. We had one overweight woman who lost only 7 pounds in the first three months, but felt so much physically better on the diet that she stuck it out. She had lost 25 pounds at the end of a year. Doesn't sound like much to some folks until you realize that this was the first time in her life she had EVER lost ANY weight no matter what she had tried, including liquid low calorie diet fasts. That 25-pound weight loss plus her feeling of well-being and great energy made her feel like a million dollars.

And finally, your body will not just keep losing weight. The diet will not make you disappear or turn into a pin-thin fashion model. For the first few weeks you may lose 2 - 3 pounds per week. Then it will slow to 1 - 2 pounds per week for a few months, then down to 1 pound a week, then 1 pound per two to three weeks. Eventually you body will find the level it wants to stay at which should be close to your ideal weight. If you were very overweight, this loss will continue until you have reduced several pounds and several belt-sizes. But if you were only a few pounds overweight, the weight loss may subside in as little as 2-3 months. And, if you are absolutely normal weight (and normal BMI) and have chosen to follow this diet for hypoglycemia or high triglycerides or known hyperinsu-linemia, remember these conditions may improve with no extra weight loss.

So know what's happening to your body. Keep the faith and keep the diet.

Chapter Ten:
Life on the G/O

Can this diet fit in with my culture?

Many people question whether any single diet is adaptable enough to fit in with the diversity of cultures that we Americans possess. We would answer this question by saying that the **Goldberg-O'Mara Diet** is a diet plan that advises you on the types of nutrients and composition of foods to eat. How you prepare them is up to your own creativity. Let us also say that the crisis of overweight Americans is not something you can blame on how your relatives taught you to cook. Many of our most famous cultural recipes are completely acceptable in the diet. Unfortunately, the desire for cheap and profitable processed foods by the food manufacturers coupled with our fast-paced society and quest for convenience foods combined to form a bad mix. Yours or anybody else's ancestors didn't give you this problem.

Consider what we actually eat on a regular basis (before you started this diet). Most Americans are eating a "low fat" breakfast of cereal made from refined flours with little or no fiber, milled flour-and-sugar breakfast pastries "enriched" with artificially added vitamins, fruit juices (maybe with artificially added calcium), and skim milk as their only protein source. Fast foods supply us with lunch and dinner. These meals consist of burgers and fries (in vegetable oils maybe, but more likely fried in those that are higher in polyunsaturated, not monounsaturated fats) or carryout pizzas and other "Americanized" Chinese, Italian, and Mexican foods. Pizzas are now prized for their excessively thick, high carbohydrate bread crusts and "low fat" cheeses. Tacos and burritos are loaded with high carbohydrate shells and fillings. So-called "Chinese" foods lie in heavily-starched sauces on piles of rice.

Snacks are high carbohydrate chips, pastries, cookies, rice cakes, and fruits. We think we're doing well if we have a salad with lunch or dinner or make our kids drink fruit juices with meals. And, of course, if we do cook at home, potatoes, pasta, and rice are the main side dishes. All those carbohydrates, and we think we're doing a great job?

Your grandparents, who are more likely to represent your cultural heritage, did not eat like this. They also did not have the weight problems we do. Let's look at some of their more traditional meals and see how we have deviated from them.

Have you ever watched an extended Chinese family order in a Chinese restaurant? Their rice is served in small side dishes that they eat in only small amounts. Their main dish is likely to be a whole fish with many sides of vegetables, simply steamed or stir-fried, without starchy sauces.

Italian cooking is a wonder and diverse depending upon the area of origination. A meal may consist of chicken, veal, or fish, large salads and vegetables. Pasta is a side dish, not the main pig-out dish we've distorted it to be.

Hispanic cuisine is as broad in scope as the geography of the countries involved. Since many of the countries have fishing access, fish and shellfish are parts of this cultural heritage. Also, highly seasoned chicken and pork dishes are featured. It is a sad commentary on our limited understanding of the variety of cuisine when we think a giant burrito stuffed with beans and cheese represents this cooking.

Creole cooking is loaded with vegetables, fish, and shellfish. New Orleans omelets are legendary. We've distorted this by placing more emphasis on the hash browns than on the main course.

French cooking is prized for its pastries and exquisite sauces. But, their pastries are usually small in size and not heavily sugared, but rather, higher in egg and butter content. We've confused having a single, small tart or cream puff for dessert once a week with mandatory desserts with EVERY dinner and even LUNCH! The French would more likely finish their evening meal with assorted cheeses.

Israeli and Arabic cooking thrive on yogurt, salads, and fish, yet in the United States, we seem to have lost these traditions. The Mediterranean areas are known for their consumption of olive oil, yet here, our meals have drifted away from olive oil in cooking and in dressing vegetables and meats. The second and third generation descendants of eastern Europe and the former USSR heritage have seem to forgotten that kefir was part of everyone's daily diet.

So, what can we do? We need to retool the kitchen, quit blaming our ancestors and re-discover our roots, so to speak.

But, we also have another problem. The above solution is not as easy as just restocking. Our live ARE complicated. We DO run constantly. We HAVE TO use convenience foods, often many times a week in order to accomplish the many things our lives demand of us. In the next few sections, we'd like to discuss what this means to each of us, women, men and kids on the G-O.

WOMEN ON THE G-O

Women are the traditional caretakers of the family. Even with the revolution in the workplace with the majority of households now having mothers who work, the business of planning meals and running the household, has remained women's work. This is not to say that men are not assuming responsibility. But, the philosophy of the household is often set by the matriarch, even if the mood is dependent upon all its members. In your household, you may have resigned yourself to the fact that you're not superwoman and that it's OK to eat out and carry-out food. Now, you need to make some choices.

Here's a typical scenario. You've worked all day. It' s five o'clock, you've got to do your grocery shopping, get home, and serve dinner (before working on next morning's presentation or taking your kid to a scout's meeting). You are in the supermarket with a list, we hope. Despite your best planning, it STILL takes a while to complete your shopping. Decision point. Do you run through the drive-up window and pick up burgers-and-fries? After all, you are exhausted by now. Your day isn't done yet. You've got all this to unpack and still another task or two to do. You could start the diet again next week, right? WRONG.

What you need to do is to have a plan ready from the time before you ever got to this point. You need to establish new habits that are as convenient for you as the old ones were. On the day that you have another thing to do after work, make sure that dinner is started and cooking while you're doing that other task. For example, have chili, stew, sausages and peppers, or a pot roast cooking in the crockpot. That way, all you need is a large salad and dinner's ready. Have chicken prepared and seasoned in a baking pan and show your son or daughter how to preheat the oven and throw it in an hour before you get home. Prior planning will reduce the chances of slipping back into old ways.

One thing that is so appealing about carry-out is that you can serve out of the cartons and throw away the mess. No clean up. Well, if you stock your house with aluminum foil, cooking bags, and canola spray (for the crockpot and casserole pans), you can still keep clean ups to a minimum. Remember too, if you have leftovers after dinner, you can take these for your lunch the next day and save money while you're improving your diet.

Another good practice to get into is to cook in advance when you do have the time. While you're chopping vegetables for one recipe, chop and freeze an extra bag or just assemble that entire second meal at the same time. If you have time to make waffles, make a double batch and freeze them for a second breakfast at a later time.

Okay, you haven't done any of the above yet and you're in that supermarket deciding whether to get carry-out or not. You still have another choice. Before you return to your old habits, head over to the deli section. Most markets have rotisserie chicken, turkey breasts and pork roasts for sale. Buy one of these, pick up a bag of premade salad and a large bag of broccoli-cauliflower-carrot medley. While you are dressing the salad, you can steam or microwave the other vegetables. If you want, you can buy a jar of premade Alfredo, hollandaise, or cheese sauce and heat it up to put on the vegetables. The cost and convenience of that dinner rivals or beats the drive-thru, yet gives you a real dinner on the G-O. Splurge and buy some sugar-free ice cream for dessert.

Dieting can be a drag for women. Most diets involve deprivation of something to which you are accustomed. In the case of the **Goldberg-O'Mara Diet**, we are not asking you to count calories or to eat funny foods. But we are asking you to adopt some new habits. Eventually, the market will catch up with the demand and we will have more appropriate and healthy convenience foods from which to choose. Right now, the market believes we want fake fat, no fat, low fat and high net carbs, so that's what they're providing. Eventually, they will come to know that we want high fiber, high monounsaturated fat, very low net carbohydrate foods. They'll come around when we stop buying the other stuff and they see the drop in sales.

OK. You walked in the door and you kids attacked the bags looking for snacks. If you had the right things on the shopping list, they could pull out some high fiber crispbread and tasty cheese spreads or peanut butter and start munching while you're getting dinner on the table. See, it's not so hard.

MEN ON THE G-O

Those men in our study thought we were kidding when we told them what was on the diet. Eat meat, fish, nuts, cheese and have a glass of wine or a light beer? No problem. Just give up potatoes and rice and chips? You're kidding me. Eat more vegetables? And I'll lose weight? You're pulling my leg.

We had to tell them to try it to believe it.

And once they did try the **Goldberg-O'Mara Diet,** the men were the easiest to convince. They were also the most impressed with their weight loss, losing the "pooch" around the middle and the "love handles" that they had carried for way too long and had accepted as middle age manhood. As the diet spread around, some of our most interesting testimonials came from men. Whoever thinks that men don't have body image issues is wrong! We heard many stories about the pride those men who lost weight felt when they ran into old buddies who hadn't seen them in a while. Their slimmed down bodies and smaller waist sizes were quickly noticed and envied!

Why is this diet so good for men? One of the main reasons the diet was so well accepted is that the diet involved little changes for men. But, the little changes had BIG impacts.

We found that most men are not particularly interested in sweets. They got their excess carbohydrates from breads and potatoes. If you can provide them with other vegetables, they will usually accept them after a bit of coaxing. If they don't get pasta for dinner, so what? They're more than happy to eat roasted chicken.

What we had to work hardest on, was to get some of our guys to accept the additional foods that they needed to make their diet nutritious. That is, they had to eat more vegetables with a greater variety than they were accustomed to eating and they had to increase monounsaturated fats and fiber and add fermented milk products to their diets. Fortunately most of them liked nuts and seeds and olive oil was fine. Even yogurt or kefir was acceptable to the majority. The key was to have these around the house all the time.

Vegetables were another story. We had some who really resisted eating vegetables. It was almost like dealing with children. In fact, when we talked with them we found that this dislike for vegetables had a life-long history attached. We found that we could get them to eat sauerkraut, coleslaw, green salad, but after that, it took some work.

They were losing weight so why did they have to eat more vegetables? This was a common question of theirs. So, this point is especially important to make once again. Anyone will lose weight on a low carbohydrate diet, BUT unless the rest of the modifications are ALSO made, the impact on your biochemistry can be hazardous. We told you earlier that up to 30% of people on one popular low carbohydrate diet had worsening of their lipid profiles, potentially increasing their cardiac risk. Following the **Goldberg-O'Mara Diet** in its entirety provides a safeguard against this occurring. And that means, increasing monounsaturated fats, increasing fiber, adding fermented milk products and eating a variety of vegetables, too!

Another point to watch for concerns the recommendations about alcohol. Studies have shown that small amounts of alcohol may have a positive benefit for people. It doesn't mean that you HAVE to drink, however. The diet provides an adequate amount of natural antioxidants in the other foods recommended. Also, if you do drink, DON'T exceed the recommended amounts per day. That is, one drink for women and up to two drinks for men per day. A drink is equivalent to one light beer, one 5 oz. glass of dry wine, or one shot of whiskey or similar alcohol. That doesn't mean you can have more if you had none for the previous three days. Drinking more than recommended will raise triglycerides and increase your cardiac risk. (Not to mention the social and other health impacts of excess drinking!)

Men are often looked upon as the "Grillmeisters" of their households. Don't ask why, just accept this cultural bias. This diet is perfect for you to show your health consciousness and culinary expertise. Why not use that grill as often as possible, with both direct and indirect cooking methods to assure the best meats, fish, and vegetables? The only warning here is regarding barbeque sauce. You'll have to experiment and make your own or find sugar-free varieties. Perhaps you'll want to cultivate more smokiness or hot-spicy tastes in your cooking and less "sugar-y" flavorings. You can create a custom sauce to meet these goals and still be on the diet. If you're making a teriyaki marinade, you can easily substitute no-calorie brown sugar sweetener into the recipe. Be creative.

Make sure you have a variety of marinated vegetable salads in the refrigerator to serve with your grilled items. The **Recipes** section offers some good suggestions. Simple sliced cucumbers, onions, and green peppers in oil and vinegar make a great salad. Remember, if they're always waiting in the refrigerator, you won't have an excuse to substitute unhealthy choices.

KIDS ON THE G-O

The **Goldberg-O'Mara Diet** has been used anecdotally in dozens of kids with success. At the time of this writing, we are collaborating with a colleague in pediatrics in the formal study of obese adolescents in her practice. Specifically, we are looking to identify the frequency of hyperinsulinemia, the lipid patterns, the waist-to-hip ratios and the responses of these and other nutritional parameters to the diet. But, there is already enough in the literature to suggest that we need to start reducing excessive amounts of carbohydrates in our children now. Especially those who are battling obesity. And, it makes good sense to start developing good eating habits in our kids now so as to avoid future problems with obesity. What kinds of things can we do?

Kids are under enormous marketing pressure to consume a variety of high net carbohydrate foods. Some common examples seen on television during children's programming include:

- cereals made from refined flours

- fruit flavored, corn syrup sweetened, starch-based snacks

- high starch, fried or baked snacks

- breakfast pastries made from refined sugars and milled flours (albiet "vitamin-enriched")

- ready-to-toast or microwave high starch and/or high sugar "hot" snacks

These items are compelling. They're often in large bright displays in the snack aisles and are often "features" at the end-of-aisle displays. The drinks that are sold to wash them down include highly sugared "juice" drinks and high carbohydrate sodas. And these are sold in increasingly-larger sizes. This is an American phenomenon. You would never see the amount of store space devoted to such items in other countries. They have not developed the American craving for sugar and the snack products made from it. And. our children are suffering from the success of this market with an epidemic of obesity and its related medical disorders. We must do something to stop this.

Granted, we can't take on the world. But, we can have an impact on our own households and upon our own children. And, as kids get older, they can make their own choices.

What about the typical lunch and after-school hangouts? They are often fast food restaurants and snack bars. And what kinds of foods are tempting the kids there? High carbohydrate french fries, candy bars, pop, and shakes. With all this pressure, is there an alternative?

Well, yes, but the kids themselves are going to have to recognize it and buy into it. Until the present market suffers losses in sales, the foods they choose to sell will be the same. Kids are going to have to bring their own lunches or find stores at lunch time in which to buy premade tuna, meat, and vegetable salads, cheese cubes, string cheese, hard boiled eggs, hot vegetable and meat soups, and yogurt. And, they'll need to wash them down with no calorie pop, iced tea, or bottled water. This isn't impossible. It's just a new choice.

Kids who are struggling with weight problems need to start eating right immediately. One of the best ways to change their patterns of eating is to do it with a buddy. If you're not the only one with a meal from home or the only one who goes to the local market instead of the snack shop at lunch, it will be easier to change. "Find a buddy" is probably the best advice we have to offer.

The general principles of the **Goldberg-O'Mara Diet** can be followed by children and adolescents, that is: No foods with excess NET carbohydrates, encourage high monounsaturated fat foods, encourage fiber, encourage a variety of vegetables, encourage fermented milk products.

What if all the kids are going to a pizza parlor? Can't my child go? Of course, but have them order the thinnest crust pizza. Put two pieces together, then discard the top crust. Bingo, you just reduced carbs by half. Diet pop and salad to accompany, of course.

What if they're all going to a hamburger joint? What can my child eat? Try a double cheeseburger and discard most of the bun while eating. No fries. Diet pop or iced tea. Feel deprived? Order a second double-cheese. This feeling of loss over the fries doesn't continue for long.

Kids will just have to avoid some fast food places which offer no healthy options at all. You can now figure out those places for yourself just by thinking of their menus. You also know what foods simply cannot be in your household: None of those items listed at the beginning of this section, no candy, no high carb snacks, no breads from milled flours, no potatoes, no pasta, no rice. Buy plenty of high fiber crispbread, peanut butter, cream cheese, string cheese, nuts and seeds, tart apples, fresh berries, plain yogurt (that you can sweeten with no calorie sweetener and berries).

Kids do have higher metabolic rates than adults. They're growing, of course. So, caloric intakes have to allow for this. Maybe they COULD cheat and get away with it? NOT LIKELY. The reason you or your child is reading this section is because you have a weight problem now. It IS very important for overweight kids to be checked out by their pediatrician or family physician before starting on a new diet. It IS possible for your child to have an endocrine problem. And, if your child has been overweight for a while, they may have a medical complication of obesity already. Their doctor can give them a thorough checkup and order appropriate testing. Then, if the doctor agrees, start the diet and let's get GO-ing.

A general reminder for all who are reading this section. You are bucking the system right now. You have been the victim of too many unhealthy food choices which have been inadvertently foisted upon the American public. But, you can change. In your household, probably most of the members are sharing a problem with obesity. After all, you're likely eating the same foods. Sometimes, the best "buddy" may be the person in your own household. If you take this return to good eating as a family challenge, you may have more success. Try it.

Postscript

At the beginning of this book, we asked you to find your personal BMI and to record it along with your weight and measurements of your waist and hips. Then we told you to put the paper with these measurements away in a drawer. If you have been on the diet for 12 weeks, it's now time to pull those measurements out and compare your present numbers with those from 12 weeks ago.

How did you do? As well as expected? Better? We told you that our study subjects lost an average of 20 pounds and 5 inches at the waist. But there was variability among the group.

If you lost less than this, maybe you didn't have that much to lose in the first place. We have found that once you approach your ideal body weight, this diet will keep you in balance. It will not make you lose more weight or become too skinny.

Or, you may have lost fat but made muscle. This could happen if you've been exercising. You may find your waist size went down (where we store our excess fat), but the pounds may not be as impressive. So what? You were out to lose fat. Muscle weighs more.

Or maybe you are taking one of the many medications that slow down your weigh loss like we talked about in Chapter Nine. You'll still get there. It will just take a little longer.

Or, maybe you found it hard to stay away from the carbohydrates. Why not try the diet again, but this time, do it with a friend or family member? It's always easier with support. Form your own little **G-O Diet** team and help each other with ways to break your old food habits and start good eating habits.

And that brings us to our final recommendation. If you have access to the Internet (if not at home, it's as near as your public library), log onto our website (www.go-diet.com). We have a "virtual" support group there with many people who are willing to share their experiences and support you in your goal.

APPENDIX ONE

Carbohydrate and Monounsaturated Fat Food List

The next two pages contain a food diary and carbohydrate and monounsaturated fat counter for your use. For convenience you should photocopy these pages and keep them with you at all times. To use the diary, you should record everything you eat and drink. This will give you two things. It will first give you a true record of what and when you eat. Most people cannot believe how much they eat until they see it in black and white. Secondly it will act as your written record to prove if certain eating patterns or certain foods help or hinder your weight loss. Keep all your diaries until you are able to judge the carbohydrate values of foods easily.

Carbohydrate and Monounsaturated fat counter :
Net Carbs = total carbs - fiber per cup

Food	g/cup	Net Carb	% Mono
Avocado Raw Florida	230	13.8	55.1
Asparagus raw	134	3.2	
Avocado Raw California	230	4.6	64.6
Bamboo shoots	131	2.4	
Beans Snap green canned solids	135	3.5	
Beef Franks (5in long x 3/4)	45g each	1.8	47.7
Beef, Ground, Lean (<21%fat)		0	42.9
Beef tenderloin lean trimmed		0	37.7
Beef Round tip trimmed all fat		0	40.9
Broccoli, Raw Chopped	88	2.7	
Brussel Sprouts	each	1	
Cabbage (Chinese (Bok Choi))	170	0.3	
Cabbage Raw (Shredded)	70	2.2	
Carrots (baby raw)	each	0.8	
Cauliflower, raw pieces	100	4	
Celery raw	120	2.4	
Cheese Cottage Uncreamed	145	2.7	26.2
Cheese Cottage Creamed	220	5.9	28.8
Cheese Cottage 1% fat	226	6.1	28.4
Cheese Brie (melted)	240	1.2	28.6
Cheese Cheddar (diced)	132	1.7	28.4
Cheese Colby (diced)	132	3.4	28.9
Cheese Cream	232	6.3	28.2
Cheese Feta (Crumbled)	150	6.2	21.7
Cheese Mozzarella part skim	112	3.1	28.3
Cheese Mozzarella Whole Milk	112	2.5	30.1
Cheese Parmesan Grated	100	3.7	29.0
Cheese Ricotta, whole milk	246	7.4	27.7
Cheese Swiss (diced)	132	4.5	26.5
Chicken breast w skin	145	0	40.9
Chicken leg	167	0	40.5
Chives Raw Chopped	1g/tsp	1.9	
Coffee Brewed w. Tap water	237	0.9	
Cranberries Raw Chopped	110	9.4	
Cream Half & Half	242	10.4	28.9
Cream Heavy whipping	238	6.7	28.9
Cream Sour Cultured	230	9.9	28.6
Cress Garden Raw	50	2.2	
Cucumber with peel, raw	104	2	
Dandelion Greens, raw	55	3.1	

Food	g/cup	Net Carb	% Mono
Egg Hardboiled whole (chopped)	136	1.5	38.5
Egg Whole Raw Large	50g each	1.2	
Eggplant raw cubed	82	3	
Endive Raw	50	0.2	
Fish Gefilte Sweet	42g/piece	3	48.2
Fish Herring Pickled	140	13.4	66.1
Frankfurter Beef each	approx. 50g	1.8	
Ginger Root .raw	2g/tsp	13	
Gooseberries, raw	150	8.9	
Grapefruit Raw	100	6.9	
Heart of Palms, canned	146	3.2	
Kohlrabi, raw	135	3.8	
Kiwifruit, store bought	91g,each	10.5	
Kale raw	67	5.4	
Leeks Lower portion,raw	89	11.0	
Lettuce,cos or romaine, raw	56	0.4	
Lettuce, iceberg, raw	55	0.4	
Melon Cantaloupe	177	13.5	
Melons, casaba	170	9.2	
Melon Honeydew	177	15	
Melon Watermelon	154	10.5	
Mung Beans, Sprouted ,raw	104	4.3	
Mushrooms, raw	70	2.5	
Nuts, Almonds Roasted, blanched	142	9.7	65.5
Nuts, brazilnuts, dried,unblanched	140	10.4	34.8
Nuts, Coconut, meat, desiccated unsweetened	8.1	4.3	
Nuts, Coconut meat, raw,shredded	80	5	4.2
Nuts, Hazelnuts, dried,chopped	115	10.6	78.4
Nuts, Macadamia oil roasted w salt	134	4.8	78.9
Nuts, Pecans, oil roasted w. salt	110	10.3	62.4
Okra, raw	100	4.4	
Onions, raw	160	10.9	
Onions, spring, raw, chopped	100	4.7	
Papaya, raw, cubed	140	11.2	
Parsley, raw	60	1.8	
Peanuts, Spanish,raw	146	9.2	44.7
Peanut Butter, Smooth w salt	258	38.2	47.0
Peppers, sweet, green, raw	149	6.9	
Peppers, sweet, red, raw	149	6.6	
Peppers, sweet, yellow, raw	149	8.0	
Pickles, cucumber, sour	155	1.6	
Pickles, cucumber, dill	143	4.2	
Plums (raw)	66	7.6	
Prickly pears, raw	149	8.9	

Food	g/cup	Net Carb	% Mono
Potato Skins (Raw)	100	9.9	
Pumpkin canned	245	12.7	
Pumpkin, Raw,cubed	116	7	
Radichio, raw	40	1.4	
Radishes, white icicle, raw	100	1.2	
Radishes, raw	116	2.3	
Raspberries. raw	123	5.9	
Rhubarb, raw	122	3.3	
Rutabaga, raw	140	7.8	
Salami Cooked Beef/slice	23	0.6	44.8
Salmon, Red Canned	369/can	0	38.4
Sardines, in tomato sauce drained	89	0	45.8
Sauerkraut Canned undrained	142	2.6	
Soy Flour Full Fat	84	20.7	21.8
Spinach Raw	30	0.2	
Squash, Summer Sliced,raw	113	2.8	
Squash, winter, raw, all varieties	116	8.5	
Squash, Spaghetti, raw	101	6.5	
Strawberries, raw	152	7.1	
Tofu, raw firm	126	2.5	22.2
Tomatillos, raw, diced	132	5.1	
Tomatoes, raw, red, ripe	180	6.3	
Tuna, White canned drained	172	0	26.7
Turnips, raw cubed	130	5.7	
Veggieburgers (Morningstar)	110	1.5	35.6
Waterchestnuts, Chinese canned	140	13.9	
Wheat bran crude	58	12.6	41.7
Yogurt Plain 8gprotein/8oz	245	11.4	27.7

My Diet Diary

Use a diary like this to keep track of what you eat and how you feel afterwards. This way you will identify the foods you are sensitive to and which cause problems with your weight loss program.

Date and Time	Food Description	Amount

Notes to myself:

Appendix Two: Glossary

Term	Meaning
Calorie	A unit of energy. It is the amount of energy required to raise one gram of water by one degree Fahrenheit. Nutritionist use the term with a capital C to mean 1000 calories or a Kilocalorie.
Carbohydrates	Nutritional term meaning compounds containing only carbon, hydrogen and oxygen. They are commonly simple sugars and bigger molecules made up by joining from two to many of the simple sugars together. Examples are glucose, lactose, sucrose, maltose, starch and glycogen. Not all carbohydrates are digestible by humans.
Cholesterol	A waxy sterol which is manufactured by all animal cells.
HDL	High Density Lipoprotein – a protein and lipid particle in the blood, which functions to remove cholesterol from cells. Higher blood levels are more desirable.
Hormone	A chemical messenger secreted by one organ which influences remote tissues.
Insulin	A hormone secreted by the pancreas.
Lactobacillus	A lactic acid producing bacterium, which is used in the manufacture of, fermented milk products. It is also a normal constituent of the intestine and the vagina.

Term	Meaning
LDL	Low Density Lipoprotein – a protein and lipid particle in the blood which carries most of the bloods cholesterol. When damaged it can be deposited in the artery wall. Lower values are more desirable.
Lipids	These are oily and waxy substances such as fats and cholesterol.
Triglycerides	Fat molecules composed of three fatty acids attached to a glycerol molecule.
VLDL	Very Low Density Lipoprotein – a protein and lipid particle in the blood whose function is to transport non-dietary triglycerides around the body. Lower blood values are more desirable.

APPENDIX THREE
Frequently Asked Questions about the Goldberg-O'Mara Diet

Alcohol
How much can I have?
It varies, but no more than one 5 oz. glass of dry wine or one small cocktail or one light beer per day for women. Up to 2 for men.

Artificial Sweeteners
Can I use them?
Yes. All artificial sweeteners are OK. You must not cook with nutrasweet. Substitute Sugar Twin or SweetOne in cooking and baking. Only buy plain or artificially sweetened yogurt or Kefir (a yogurt like drink) diet sodas or mixers or make them yourself. Packets have 1 gram carbs each. Tablets and liquids have zero carbs.

Brans –Flax
Where can I buy wheat or other brans and flax seeds?
Most healthfood store and specialty sections of large food stores. Grind the flax seeds in your coffee grinder.

Caffeine
Can I take caffeine drinks?
Yes. But keep it to a minimum. Caffeine is a diuretic and causes water loss. This can lead to headaches.

Calories
Do I have to count Calories?
No. Your own body will control intake and appetite on this diet. Your calorie intake reduces to normal amounts.

Cholesterol
Will eating all that fat increase my cholesterol?
No. In most cases it will reduce your cholesterol. If you do see a rise, this may be brought back down with garlic and vitamin E supplements. The emphasis on monounsaturated fats and fiber in this diet are the key features to prevent cholesterol from rising.

Constipation
Will this diet be constipating?
No. After the first week we emphasize both soluble and insoluble fibers intake and yogurt or Kefir. This will bulk the stool. Also take at least 6-8 glasses of total liquids per day.

Diabetes

I have diabetes. Is the diet safe?

That question is being answered by current research. Consult with your doctor.

Exercise

Do I have to exercise?

Not until you can. Consult with your physician.

Fiber

What is fiber?

That's the indigestible carbohydrates of plants. Rich sources are nuts, veggies, psyllium, brans and flaxseeds.

Headaches

Why do I get them?

Headaches are normal in the first two to three days as you body adjusts. After that it is usually a sign of dehydration. Drink more fluids.

How Long

How long must I stay on the diet?

As long as it takes. Never go back to what you are doing now. That's what got you into trouble. You may have to eat this way for the rest of your life. Only you will be able to decide.

Hunger

Will I be hungry?

Probably not. This diet produces natural hunger suppressants. Never go hungry. Eat low carb snacks to tide you over.

Ketones

Is Ketosis dangerous?

No. It's a natural state after fasting or exercise. The diet forces it to be your normal state.

Is Ketosis the same as ketoacidosis?

No. Ketoacidosis is a dangerous condition associated with Type 1 diabetes. It has nothing to do with this diet.

Do I have to test my urine with ketostix?

No. Testing for ketosis is not the objective. Weight loss is.

Kidney disease
Will low carbohydrate dieting give me kidney disease?
No. There are no studies showing a low carbohydrate diet can actually cause kidney damage.

Low Carbohydrate Diet
Why do you lose weight on a low carb diet?
Control of insulin is the basis of all low carb diets. By forcing the body to burn fats for fuel you waste calories. The higher fat delays stomach emptying. Your snacking and appetite cravings go down. Your calorie intake normalizes.

Psyllium
What is Psyllium?
It is the husk of a grass seed. Buy Sugar free flavored or plain Metamucil. Use it in wheat bran pancakes, meatballs or drink it in club soda.

Recipes
Where can I find them?
We will be publishing a book. Also look on the internet and in the bookstores for low carbohydrate cookbooks. Check frequently with our website at http://www.go-diet.com

Snacks
Are snacks allowed?
Yes, so long as they are low carbohydrate snacks like chicken wings, jerky, cheese or macadamia nuts, low carb veggies with dips, pork rinds, hard-boiled eggs.

Triglycerides
Will all that fat increase my blood triglycerides?
No. Most high blood triglycerides are caused by carbohydrate ingestion. Almost all people will lower their serum triglycerides when eating the G/O Diet(c) way

Vegetarianism

Can I be vegetarian?

Yes, but it will be pretty boring. You cannot eat excess fruits or legumes or pastas that are the heart of the variety for vegetarians. Vegans do not do well on this type of diet. Lacto-Ovo-vegetarians can do very well with cheeses and texturized soy products.

Weight Loss

How fast will I lose weight?

Varies for each individual and how strict you are at cutting carbohydrates. It may vary for one to three pounds per week after the initial rapid weight loss until you reach your target weight.

Acknowledgements

The authors would like to acknowledge the patience and support of their families throughout this project. Without their continued encouragement, this project would have been much more difficult to complete.

We would also like to acknowledge the assistance of summer research student, Kevin Krembs. We acknowledge the study subjects who bravely tolerated many weigh-ins and laboratory tests. The study subjects and Kevin made quite a team; we all learned many things about clinical research in this process and we extend our thanks to them.

REFERENCES

DIET COMPOSITION AND RISK OF CORONARY ARTERY DISEASE

Lamarche BL, Tchernof A et al, Fasting insulin and Apolipoproein B levels and low density lipoprotein particle size as risk factors for ischemic heart disease. Journal of the American Medical Association 1998 ; 279: 1955-61.

Maron DJ; Fair JM; Haskell WL. Saturated fat intake and insulin resistance in men with coronary artery disease. Circulation, 1991, 84:5, 2020-7

Stampfer MJ, Krauss RM, et al. A prospective study of triglyceride level, low density particle diameter and risk of myocardial infarction. Journal of the American Medical Association .1996: 276: 882-888

DIET COMPOSITION AND SERUM LIPIDS

Adler A and Holub BJ. Effect of garlic and fish-oil supplementation on serum lipid and lipoprotein concentrations in hypercholesterolemic men. American Journal of Clinical Nutrition 1997; 65: 445-50

Knoop RH, Walden CE et al, Long-term cholesterol lowering effects of 4 fat restricted diets in hypercholesterolemic and combined hyperlipidemic men, Journal of the American Medical Association, 1997; 278: 1509-1515

DIET COMPOSITION AND WEIGHT LOSS

Golay A, Allaz A, Morel Y et al, Similar weight loss with low- high-carbohydrate diets, American Journal of Clinical Nutrition 1996; 63: 174-8

Goldberg JM, O'Mara K and Krembs K, Effect of a high monounsaturated fat, very low carbohydrate diet on weight and serum lipids. Clinical Chemistry 1998: 44(S6): A158

DIET COMPOSITION AND WOMEN'S HEALTH
Cohen L, Zhao Z, Zang A, Tin T. Wynn B, Rivenson A, Mammary Tumorigenesis in F344 Rats--Journal of the National Cancer Institute 1996; 88:13

Franceschi S, Favero A, Intake of macronutrients and risk of breast cancer. Lancet 1996; 347(9012):1351-6

Jeppesen J, Schaaf P et al, Effects of low fat, high carbohydrate diets on risk factors for ischemic heart disease in posrmenopausal women, American Journal of Clinical Nutrition 1997; 65: 1027-1033

Nicklas BJ, Katzel LI ,et al. Effects of an American Heart Association diet and weight loss on lipoprotein lipids in obese, posmenopausal women. American Journal of Clinical Nutrition 1997; 66: 853-9

Rexrode K, Hennekens C, Willett W, et al, A prospective study of body mass index, weight change and risk of stroke in women. Journal of the American Medical Association, 1997; 227:19, 1539-1545

Rexrode K, Carey V, Hennekens C, et al, Abdominal adiposity and coronary heart disease in women. Journal of the American Medical Association 1998; 280:21, 1843-1848

Stoll B. Timing of weight gain in relation to breast cancer risk. Annals of Oncology1995; 6: 245-248

EFFECT OF FOODS ON IMMUNITY
Schiffrin EJ, Brassart D, Servin AL, Rochat, F and Donnet-Hughes A. Immune modulation of blood leukocytes in humans by lactic acid bacteria. American Journal of Clinical Nutrition 1977; 66: 515S - 520S

Solis-Pereya B, Aattouri N and Lemonnier D. Role of food in the stimulation of cytokine production. American Journal of Clinical Nutrition 1977; 66: 521S

EFFECT OF MONOUNSATURATED FATS ON DIABETES

Campbell L, Marmot P, Dyer J, et al, The high monounsaturated fat diet as a practical alternative for NIDDM. Diabetes Care 1994: 17:3, 177-182

Garg A, High monounsaturated fat diets for patients with diabetes mellitus: a meta-analysis. American Journal of Clinical Nutrition 1998; 67(suppl): 577S-582S

Low C, Grossman E, Gumbiner B, Potentiation of effects of weight loss by monounsaturated fatty acids in obese NIDDM patients. Diabetes 1996; 45: 569-575

HYPERINSULINEMIA/ INSULIN RESISTANCE

Folsom AR; Ma J; McGovern PG; Eckfeldt H. Relation between plasma phospholipid saturated fatty acids and hyperinsulinemia. Metabolism 1996, 45:2, 223-228

Grey N and Kipnis D. Effect of diet composition on the hyperinsulinemia of obesity. New England Journal of Medicine 1971; 285:15, 827-831

Modan M, Halkin H, Almog S, et al, Hyperinsulinemia- a link between hypertension, obesity, and glucose intolerance. Journal of Clinical Investigation 1985; 75: 809-817

Moller D and Flier J. Insulin resistance- mechanisms, syndromes, and implications. New England Journal of Medicine 1991; 325:13, 938-948

O'Mara K, Shah U, Goldberg J, Krembs K, Prevalence of hyperinsulinemia in obese subjects presenting for a weight loss program. Chest 1997; 112 (3) Suppl.: 76S

Solymoss B, Marcil M, Chaour M, et al, Fasting hyperinsulinism, insulin resistance syndrome, and coronary artery disease in men and women. The American Journal of Cardiology, 1995; 76: 1152-1156

Zimmet P, Hyperinsulinemia-how innocent a bystander? Diabetes Care 1993; 16(supplement 3): 56-70

PEDIATRICS AND ADOLESCENTS

Caprio S, Bronson M, et al., Coexistence of severe insulin resistance and hyperinsulinemia in preadolescent obese children, Diabetologia 1966; 39:1489-1497

Dennison BA, Rockwell HL and Baker MS, Excess fruit juice consumption by preschool-aged children is associated with short stature and obesity. Pediatrics 1997; 99: 15-22

Division of Health Examination Statistics, Centers for Disease Control. "Update: Prevalence of overweight among children, adolescents, and adults- United States, 1988-1994" in Journal of the American Medical Association, 1997; 227:14, 1111

Steinberger J, Moorehead C, Katch V, Rocchini A, Relationship between insulin resistance and abnormal lipid profile in obese adolescents. The Journal of Pediatrics, 1998 126:5, 690-695

Willi SM, Oexmann MJ, Wright NM, Collop NA and Key, Jr LL, The effects of a high protein, low-fat, ketogenic diet on adolescents with morbid obesity: body chemistries and sleep abnormalities. Pediatrics 1998; 101: 61-7

A

alfredo sauce 84
almond macaroons 76
almonds 24,62,76,77
antioxidants 12
atherosclerosis 6, 7, 60

B

beef 12, 16, 24, 25, 61, 65, 66, 68
blood clots 7
BMI 5, 11, 12, 29, 30, 51
bran 19, 23, 25, 31, 47, 62, 63, 65, 68, 69, 71, 72, 74, 75
breads 74, 75, 76, 77, 78
broccoli soup 79

C

caesar's dressing 85
caffeine 34
calcium 22
caloric restriction 5, 6
calories 5, 6, 7, 8, 12, 15, 31, 37, 49, 57, 59, 105, 106, 125
cancer 45, 46, 47, 48, 134
Candida albicans 48
canola 12, 14, 17, 18, 61, 71, 101
carbohydrate 12, 13, 14, 17, 21, 26, 32, 33, 34, 35, 36, 39, 40, 42, 44, 45, 49, 50, 52, 60, 69, 72, 119, 125, 134, 135
carbohydrates 12, 13, 14, 17, 21, 26, 32, 33, 34, 35, 36, 39, 40, 42, 44, 45, 49, 50, 52, 60, 69, 72, 119, 125, 134, 135
cheese 15, 16, 17, 18, 19, 26, 48, 62, 63, 66, 67, 68, 69, 70, 72, 75, 78, 79, 80, 81, 84, 85, 90, 91, 92, 94, 100, 101, 102, 106

cheese omelet 100
chicken 12, 14, 16, 17, 18, 19, 24, 25, 26, 63, 66, 67, 68, 69, 101, 102
chocolate cheesecake 78
chocolates 80
cholesterol 1, 6, 19, 30, 31, 32, 35, 36, 38, 39, 40, 41, 44, 45, 47, 49, 50, 53, 125, 126, 134
coconut and almond 77
cold float 99
constipation 31, 47
coronary artery disease 6, 7, 44, 50, 133
cream 26, 43, 68, 69, 73, 75, 78, 79, 80, 84, 88, 89, 90, 96, 99, 100

D

Dairy 17
diaries 119

E

EGGPLANT LASAGNA 81
eggs 16, 17, 24, 26, 62, 67, 69, 71, 72, 74, 75, 84, 88, 89, 90, 91, 93, 94, 95, 96, 100, 101
exercise 1, 3, 5, 11, 32, 36, 39, 53, 57

F

fasting 29, 30, 35, 39, 46
fat 1, 11, 17, 26, 29, 32, 34, 35, 36, 38, 39, 41, 42, 43, 44, 45, 47, 49, 50, 51, 52, 72, 84, 119, 120, 133, 134, 135
fatty acids 17, 32, 43, 45, 46, 136

Check our Web Pages Frequently for the Latest Updates and Offers

http://www.go-diet.com

Order additional copies of this book direct from the publisher.

I would like to order
___ **copies of the GO-Diet @ $19.95 each**   _____

Illinois Residents add 8.5% ($1.70) per book_____

Add $5.00 Shipping and Handling per book _____

Total amount enclosed (U.S. Funds only)   _____

Make checks or MO payable to GO Corp
P.O. Box 48026
Niles, IL 60714

Ship to

Name_____

Address_____

City, State, Zip_____

Please allow 2-4 weeks for delivery